Ashtanga Yoga
Stories from Beyond the Mat

Jason Stein

Ashtanga Yoga: Stories from Beyond the Mat

Copyright © 2011 by Jason Stein

Cover photo © 2009 by Kelly Lynn Hubert

All rights reserved. All wrongs reversed. Savor the luminosity. No part of this book may be reproduced in any form by any electronic or mechanical means including photocopying, recording, or information storage and retrieval without permission in writing from the author.

Printed in U.S.A

ISBN: 978-1467949989

ISBN-13: 1467949981

www.leapinglanka.blogspot.com

Email: leapinglanka@gmail.com

DEDICATION

To Tim Miller and, through him, Pattabhi Jois.

I owe much of what is good, true and beautiful in my life to the practice of Yoga that they have taught.

Any "tragedies of small enlightenment" are my own.

CONTENTS

DEDICATION	I
CONTENTS	III
ACKNOWLEDGMENTS	V
INTRODUCTION	1
SHANE	5
YOGA AND NATURE	8
HOW TO GET TO MYSORE IN TWO EASY STEPS	10
THE ETERNAL RETURNING	13
MYSORE FAQ	14
MYSORE GUILT	21
MY SIDDHIS	24

A LETTER TO THE EDITOR OF *YOGA JOURNAL*	26
AGE 19	28
EXPRESSWAY TO FLEXIBILITY	31
YOU KNOW IT AIN'T EASY	33
SHANKARA AND BANDHAS	35
WHAT FIRST SERIES TAUGHT ME	37
HIMSA	39
IMBALANCES	41
YOGA ROUTINE, ENCINITAS 2002	45
FLENSING	47
WHAT I KNOW ABOUT YOGA AND FOOD	51
SUBMIT TO PRACTICE	54
RAMESH BALSEKAR IN MUMBAI	56
HOW TO MAKE ASHTANGA VINYASA MORE DIFFICULT	59

ASHTANGA YOGA JOURNAL EDIT MEETING NOTES
64

YANAL CONTROL 66

SARTORIAL SPLENDOR 68

RHIZOMATIC ASHTANGA 72

LILLIAN 74

ASHTANGA AT ALTITUDE 76

MYSORE 2005 79

GOA 2008 84

TAKE REST! 91

BLOG RESPONSE 96

BURN TO SHINE 101

THANK GOD FOR BOREDOM 102

YOGA PHOTO DUKKHA 103

BOREDOM AGAIN 107

MY LATEST PROJECTS	109
SHANKARA VERSUS DOGEN	112
ASHTANGA AND CROSSFIT	115
YOUR UNIVERSE	124
MY LEAST FAVORITE POSE	127
HOW TO GET SIX-PACK ABS WITH ASHTANGA	130
YOGA TEACHER CONTRACT RIDER	133
PAIN, SUFFERING, ET AL	136
HOW TO DO ASHTANGA AND CROSSFIT	139
WHITE ELEPHANT VERSUS TERMITE PRACTICE	142
MYSORE FLASHBACKS	145
LIVING TRADITION	147
HOW TO START A MYSORE PROGRAM	150
ABOUT THE AUTHOR	158

ACKNOWLEDGMENTS

Thank you David Kennedy for the bike rides, which were not about the bike rides.

Thank you Sheenon Olson and Nate Denver for the relentless encouragement.

And of course, thank you to Tara, my delicate flower, for never accepting less than my best, and for the ferocious love and tenderness.

INTRODUCTION

This whole project started spontaneously and organically way back in 2002, when I worked a cube job that entailed heaps of writing. I would recharge between bouts of advertising and promotional drudgework by writing about my practice of Ashtanga Vinyasa and whatever else came into my head, which, over time, came to be quite strongly influenced by this practice.

This venting was published on a blog called "Leaping Lanka," which is still active at leapinglanka.blogspot.com. I named the site after Hanuman, among whose many epithets is Lankabhayankaram, the "leaper of Lanka."

Hanuman, a character from that epic myth the *Ramayana*, was for some reason an incredibly compelling character to me. Sure, Rama and Sita were, for the most part, the main protagonists in the story — and yet the action in several key parts was driven by Hanuman, this strange human-like monkey (or monkey-like human).

Hanuman contained within him the power to shake the universe, and yet had to be reminded of this fact. He moved with virtuosity between his limited, temporary form and his divine essence. He was humble and devoted and sought to avoid conflict, yet did not shy away from it when it became inevitable. He could assume whatever size the situation called for, large or small, and he was that force of reunification in constant movement between and among Rama, the epitome of divine, conditional love, and his kidnapped wife Sita, the epitome of divine, unconditional love. His was a ferocious sweetness, love and devotion.

To me, Hanuman was (and is) the ultimate yogi.

With my site thus named, I began publishing. Internet writing was interesting, for sure — I would blast off whatever percolated in my head, perhaps receive a comment or two (on a busy day), and that was it.

Flash-forward 10 years. I have the brilliant idea to compile my favorite posts and self-publish them as a book. Suddenly the gravity of the situation turns the process into a ponderous, anxious mess.

I wasn't nervous about putting my thoughts and opinions regarding Ashtanga Yoga on paper or on the Internet. No, I was nervous about publishing them. Part of my trepidation arose from my awareness that Ashtanga Vinyasa Yoga is descended from a tradition of Hindu Brahmin lineage-holders, men who strove to remove their personalities from their teachings in order to present, as Pierre-Sylvain Filliozat says, "the whole of their knowledge."

Meanwhile I've got a collection of writings that are essentially *nothing but* a collection of my individual, limited and conditional understandings of the Ashtanga Vinyasa practice.

What to do?

To back up for a second, I've practiced this style of Yoga since 1998 with equal parts fascination, obsession, passion, and love. A buddy of mine, a teacher of Ashtanga Vinyasa (who shall remain nameless!), used to exclaim, "This shit really works!" Because it did, and it does. When I found this practice it was like coming home. This was my path through the forest.

Knowing that, the question became: What now? How did I do this practice and have a family and friendships, a career, as well as take part in culture and society? I had no idea how to rejigger my life around the Yoga, or shape the Yoga around my life. I had no family members with Yoga experience, no mentors, and when I mentioned it to my friends, they looked at me like I was an alien, because unless there was beer, skateboards, girls, or videogames involved, and not necessarily in that order, the topic was pretty much off radar.

There was no sub-section in the bookstore, and truth be told, most Yoga-related bookstores reeked of patchouli, were packed with crystals, and tinkled with wind-chimes — they were, in short, for New Agers and hippies. *New Agers and hippies*?! Fuck that.

Still, as I continued to practice, I scoured these and many other bookstores and found the books on Yoga history, philosophy, and anatomy (both subtle and gross), as well as asana mechanics. I found the books of discussions, talks, lectures and darshans as well as the Yoga-related myths, Hindu and Buddhist, and the epics, great and small.

As (Saint) Morrissey once said, "the music that they constantly play, it says nothing to me about my life." Here were all these fantastic books of Yogic wisdom, knowledge, and devotion. Yet where were the books in which I could recognize my life, family, work, culture?

Thankfully, I've always kept journals, and, as I kept practicing, they were where I wrote about my relationship to and understanding of Yoga. It was through journaling that I could write about a world informed by Yoga practice, and in turn a Yoga practice informed by the world.

And so, way back in 2002, I took this journaling online on Leaping Lanka. *Ashtanga Yoga: Stories from Beyond the Mat* has been compiled from its stories, essays, sketches, and fragments. Every piece has been reworked, and in many cases entirely rewritten, for inclusion here. The very processes of writing, selecting, editing and finally publishing this book is the latest in a series of waves that are my deepening practice of Ashtanga. My own understanding and practice of Ashtanga Vinyasa Yoga has evolved to encompass a connection and intimacy, not only to Self, but also to family, friends, and culture.

During the organization of this book I also had the realization that I'm not presenting the "totality of a tradition."

The careful inclusion of both the anti-hippie sentiment as well as the f-bomb should be a tip-off that this isn't a textbook, a guidebook, a practice manual, or a treatise on Ashtanga as a system of philosophy or soteriology.

When you read what follows, I hope that you'll see small reflections of your own experience practicing this Yoga. Just as importantly, I hope you'll also see where our experiences and perspectives differ. Just as this practice has deepened and enriched my appreciation of non-separation, it's also helped me savor our vital differences.

It's my hope the collection that follows enriches your ability to savor, too.

SHANE

Shane was tall, taller than me at 6-foot-3, his thinning hair swept up in a rockabilly pompadour and his boyish good looks slowly losing ground to the encroaching fat. He would show up at Ahimsa Yoga in San Francisco wearing white V-neck T-shirts, and he always smelled strongly and pleasantly of coffee. I want to say he had several Sailor Jerry flash-style tattoos, too, the pin-up girls, swallows, stars, and hearts reminiscent of 1940's funny pages, the ink on his skin bright and optimistic with that mix of pulp-color brilliance and nostalgia.

I came to know Shane when I first committed to a daily morning Mysore practice, a transition that had jimmied open a new perspective on Ashtanga Vinyasa Yoga. A morning practice also introduced me to a new cast of characters: the morning shift. After several years attending evening classes and becoming familiar with those regulars, to meet an entire batch of new, heretofore unseen people was like discovering some hidden tribe living right in my midst.

Tiffany and I were living in the Mission District, in a slant-floored firetrap on 27th and Guerrero. Its amenities included pungi-spike splinters and an uncountable and ever-changing mass of illegals sleeping on sweat-stained mattresses in the building's common basement. On weekends the small, sun-darkened men would drink cases of beer and listen to what sounded like Mexican polka music, the bomp-bomp of the drum and the whine of accordion turned up full volume. I never felt in any physical danger, but in our neighborhood the men on the street would hiss, suck, and sometimes grab at Tiffany, so I was in constant fear of what the men in the basement, galvanized by those cases of beer, might do.

The studio, Ahimsa Yoga, was just three blocks away on foot. The space was tucked between a grocery and a storefront church, and Alice, the owner, had turned it into a warm and inviting Yoga studio. She is a short, hyperintelligent woman with a fierce full-back tattoo of Kali done by the famous tattoo artist Ed Hardy. It was full-on Kali, too: tongue protruding, garland necklace of bloody severed heads, one hand holding a bloody dagger, the other a severed head. Alice could be just as intense.

This was where I met Shane. He was gregarious, friendly, and quick to laugh. He was inconstant in morning practice because, as I found out, he was a member of the dockworker's union, and a few mornings a week he would head to the union office to put his number in the lottery for a day's work. The job sounded hard and exhausting. But when he could, Shane would show up on the mat, crack a few jokes, and sweat and groan his way through a Mysore practice. The sweating and groaning were both tendencies we shared.

Months passed. Tiffany and I moved out of our firetrap and into a better apartment in order for our relationship to better unravel. I returned to Encinitas. Alice closed Ahimsa.

Shane joined a long and still-growing list of people about whom I idly wonder, people I only ever knew in passing, and a few with whom I never exchanged a word. Yet in a Mysore class I was profoundly intimate with and connected to all them. We saw each other every single day, six days a week, for months on end, all of us sweaty and half-naked, moments of poise and grace alternating with shaky struggling and ragged vulnerability.

I hope Shane still practices Yoga. Maybe he's still waiting at the union office for his number to pop up. Maybe he's driving forklifts and hauling crates on the Oakland dock, his hair a bit thinner, face a bit fuller, but still with bright tattoos beaming, quick to smile and fast with a joke.

YOGA AND NATURE

During the halcyon days of my Corporate Job, my coworkers discovered I had made multiple trips to India to practice Yoga. Suddenly they assumed I preferred hemp pants, patchouli, and puka shell necklaces. They would send me emails when their cousin had a 70's VW bus for sale, or if they had extra tickets to a Phish show, or worse, a lesser-known jam band. I got invited on myriad hikes and backpacking trips.

I love practicing Yoga, don't get me wrong. But man, I hate nature. By "nature," I mean mountains, forests, the woods generally and trees specifically, creeks, brooks, streams, rivers and lakes, trails, and meadows. Flowers are okay as long as they're safely in vases and grass is acceptable as long as that shit is manicured.

Okay, really it's not so much nature itself that I hate. It's the recreational activities that surround it: hiking, climbing, camping, hunting, fishing, bird watching, tracking, ultimate Frisbee, hackee-sack, and stick tossing. Pretty much any endeavor that involves brown boots, a puffy jacket, and a stout staff.

I suppose, then, that it's fitting I live in Portland, Oregon, which is essentially a city built among a vast forest of trees that insist on crowding over every street and house, building and sidewalk, in order to cast black shadows that whisper of a primordial darkness. Portland is also just a few miles from mountains, streams, trails, hills, and valleys. In other words, you can't throw a Styrofoam coffee cup anywhere here without hitting the Great Fucking Outdoors.

I prefer urban nature: the overgrown vacant lot en route to the coffee shop; the yellow strobe of dandelions thrust between the cracks in pavement; red flowers in a white bucket sold on a freeway on-ramp; a sculpted green shrub leaning well away from the sidewalk. Acceptable wildlife includes squirrels, pigeons, cats, mid-sized dogs, and any other animal less than half my bodyweight and that, were it to go rabid, I could reliably stomp to death.

What's really at stake here? I'm scraping against the unfortunate reality that "Yoga" and "hippie" as well as "nature" are all so intimately related in peoples' minds they may as well be the same thing. The solution? Shave my head, wear all black clothing, get more tattoos … and, when people ask, tell 'em, "Nature? I hate that shit."

HOW TO GET TO MYSORE IN TWO EASY STEPS

One: buy the plane ticket.
Two: go.
Parental freak-outs, vaccinations and immunizations, the Yoga, transportation, accommodation ... the rest is incidental. There're tons of Yoga-specific advice on those subjects on various forums, blogs and Web sites, and there're general India travel suggestions and advice on-line as well as in all the travel books.[1]

Interestingly, once I reached India, used India travel guides such as Lonely Planet's seemed to be a Rupee-a-dozen at the book swaps in hostels, hotels and restaurants that catered to Westerners, such as the many I found in Mysore and Goa.

Probably the most unique tip on getting to Mysore I can offer — and which is completely obvious, and what's more, is applicable to all facets of life — is this: transcend lottery mentality.

---

1 ProTip: Save yourself money, and rather than purchase those travel books, visit large corporate bookstores with a notebook and take copious notes.

In my case, I came to the realization that I could no longer wait for money to fall out of the sky and into my lap in order to make my trip happen. I could no longer make the fulfillment of my dream to travel to India contingent on the acquisition of some abstract and nebulous "thing," in this case money. As the crusty tow-truck driver once said to me: "Wish in one hand, shit in the other, see which fills first."

First, I clarified my intentions. Then I established specific goals, built an infrastructure to sustain those goals, and acted on an earning strategy. Finally, I watered with frequent attention the garden I'd planted.

As they say, "Begin with the end in mind." In this case, I knew exactly where I wanted to end up — in Mysore, India, practicing Yoga at the Ashtanga Yoga Research Institute (now the Jois Yoga Shala). You'd be surprised, though, by how many people never make it that far, and therefore traveling to India, or Europe, or South America, or anywhere, remains an amorphous dream.

Now I had an explicit pole star around which to orbit. My dream to travel to Mysore became a goal. I had just reduced all future decisions to a blindingly simple yes/no question: will this help me travel to Mysore?

So how did I earn the money? I was pretty leveraged when it came to my monthly take-home income, so this is when I tapped into all my gifts and assets. What could I sell on Craig's List or eBay? Could I organize bake sales, garage sales, or sell my designer shoe collection at consignment stores? Could I organize knitting workshops or Olympic weight-lifting seminars? Could I charge for "freelance IT work," which could be as simple as synching my friends' iTunes?

For my first trip to Mysore, I saved paycheck money and I also sold comic books on eBay. Now, don't get me wrong: I love the shit out of comic books. But I'd been lugging around longboxes of the damn things for 15 years.

So I bundled together runs of issues, like Grant Morrison's run on *Doom Patrol*, and put 'em on eBay. That way I prevented people from cherry-picking my collection, or taking single issues and leaving the bones, and I brought in more money than if I'd sold my collection at a specialty shop. My point is, find your own personal Grant Morrison run on *Doom Patrol*.

I took refuge in the realization that I had developed the inner resources to get out of bed to make it to morning Mysore class every day. There is never going to be the "perfect" time, and you will never have the "right" amount of money. Your parents will always freak out, the car will always need new brakes, and there are always 40-minute commutes to cubicles in well-manicured office parks.

THE ETERNAL RETURNING

Why do I return to Encinitas? After all, at a certain point, usually after 7 or 8 years, one has achieved a workmanlike competency in one's chosen craft. That's roughly the length of an apprenticeship in many trades, and seems to correlate with skill acquisition, whether blowing glass, playing an instrument, speaking a foreign language, or as Patanjali has it, "Desha bandhas cittasya dharana," fixing one's attention on one thing for long periods of time.

"What you do speaks so loud that I cannot hear what you say," said Emerson. The silence that emanates from Tim Miller is so loud and so still, and reaches into such a deep place in me, that speech is superfluous, in fact futile.

I don't go for adjustments or new poses, or, I'm ashamed to admit, to even really practice asana. I return to Encinitas to see Tim Miller not "to learn his words of wisdom," to paraphrase a Hasidic rabbi, "but to see how he ties and unties his shoes."

MYSORE FAQ

Here's a morning Mysore FAQ I cobbled together for people considering making the jump. I wrote this to answer the common questions I was receiving from people considering coming to Mysore class. I also wrote it as a way to communicate my expectations and my current understanding of Mysore-style practice.

People travel a varied path on their way to a Mysore-style Ashtanga Vinyasa Yoga practice. Where do you fall on the continuum below?

1. Sporadic Led Classes
You go to class when you feel like it, and when you have the time.

2. Scheduled Led Classes
You go to led classes on a set schedule, e.g. every Monday, Thursday, and Saturday.

3. Scheduled Morning Mysore
You attend morning Mysore class on a set schedule, like every Monday, Wednesday and Friday.

4. Daily Morning Mysore
You hit class every morning but moon days and holidays.

Generally, priorities change depending on the seasons. People tend to bail on classes during the dog days of summer and during holidays.

More than just the weather, the seasons of life also affect one's capacity for Yoga asana practice. I find young adults have a difficult time committing to a schedule because generally their life-stage is characterized by heavy flux.

Also, as equally important as the season of life, your capacity for a consistent Yoga practice will vary depending on the stability of your life's big foundations, some of which are (in no particular order) home, family, health and career. Those foundations can be pretty rattled by instances such as the birth of a child, a move to a new house or new city, a relationship meltdown, or a gnarly bout of mono.

If you're somewhere between numbers 3 and 4 above, you may be considering attending a Mysore class. I teach several led Ashtanga Vinyasa classes in the evenings, but I generally resist strong-arming people into coming to Mysore. Still, at a certain point, you'll exhaust the led class setting, and that's when a Mysore class is the next stage in practice.

What Is A Mysore Class?
A Mysore-style class is a specific way of teaching and practicing Yoga within the Ashtanga Vinyasa tradition.

Students learn and practice at their own pace poses from among the several Ashtanga Vinyasa series. The postures in the sequences flow together using a special breath-movement technique called vinyasa.

The instructor teaches each sequence, pose by pose, to each student. Students practice up to the posture that is appropriate for their experience and physical capacity. The subsequent postures and series are then given as strength, flexibility and stamina improve.

It is an utterly unique Yoga class setting as the room is silent but for the sound of the breath. Students follow their own inhale-exhale and thereby move at their own pace. They can remain in poses longer, or repeat them to address "interesting" areas.

The instructor therefore tailors unique alignment adjustments as well as physical assistance to each person. In this way, each student is met where they are at each moment.

Both experienced and beginning students practice together in the same space.

The Mysore style also helps each person nurture an independent and intimate personal Yoga practice. Ultimately, you move to the rhythm of your very own breath and ability.

The Ashtanga Vinyasa method is intended as a daily practice, and traditionally takes place every day except for Saturdays and new or full moon days.

Why Is It Called "Mysore?"

This style — that of a personal Yoga practice, yet one supported amongst a like-minded gathering — originated in the south Indian city of Mysore. This method of teaching flourished under the auspices of the late Sri K. Pattabhi Jois, who helped pioneer and maintain it.

Jois taught this system for more than 60 years. He passed in 2009, and his grandson Sharath currently directs the Jois Ashtanga Yoga Institute in Mysore, India.

Is It Called Mysore Because It Makes You Sore?

It is not called Mysore because it makes you sore. Although you may experience some soreness.

Will I Get Adjusted?

I often provide hands-on adjustments to provide accurate alignment and form; I also give them to take you deeper in poses. Please let me know if you don't wish to receive any adjustments. Also, if you need help with a particular asana, don't hesitate to ask or catch my attention.

I'm A Beginner — Is Mysore For Me?

Absolute beginners are welcome! A Mysore class is perhaps the best way to learn Ashtanga Vinyasa. You can be taught individually, pose by pose, in order to establish a firm foundation, and the sequences can be scaled up or down specifically to meet your unique needs. You'll meet your limits, and yet won't sail past them.

New students are welcome to watch class before joining. If you have little to no previous Yoga experience and wish to participate, I require a Beginner's Pass, which asks for a commitment of four classes in one month.

We will begin with Surya Namaskara A, and then add Surya Namaskara B. Initially your practice will be less than 30 minutes, but in time we'll add poses, and your practice will lengthen as we introduce the standing poses and new asanas as appropriate.

Postures are given, one by one, in a prescribed, sequential order. If you have trouble with a particular posture, I can offer you a modification that is consistent with the intention of the practice.

To learn the poses "one by one" also means that, once you are given a new posture, you practice the sequence through until you get to that posture, then wind down your practice with backbends (if appropriate) and the finishing sequence. I can help you with the next posture in the sequence when it is appropriate.

Do I Have to Remember All the Poses?

If you've been to my led Ashtanga Vinyasa classes, don't worry, you'll remember more than you think!

It's definitely okay to come to Mysore class if you haven't memorized the exact poses and sequence. Just show up, make an honest effort, and then relax. Consistency is the mother of skill.

Also remember that every single person in the room, myself included, has been in your position. In a Mysore class, it's expected and okay to ask for assistance, especially if you're not clear about the next asana or correct vinyasa.

For a short period of time, you'll make a concession as you transition to a Mysore class from led classes — you'll relinquish the comfort of dependence. You've been a passenger in many led classes. You've been guided through an entire, familiar sequence. Now you're scooting into the driver's seat. Initially your practice will be shorter, and yet much more profound, as intimate as your own breath.

You will practice the sequence of poses that you can remember, no more and no less, and then, when you lose the thread, you'll move to a finishing sequence. This is when either you are exhausted and spent, or you no longer remember the next pose. These terminal points differ for each person. Given consistent effort, you will very quickly learn the sequence.

Can I Use A Cheat Sheet?

To learn the correct sequence of poses is to participate in the Ashtanga Vinyasa tradition. It's also a profound way to take charge of your own Yoga practice.

You're more than welcome to study printouts of the sequence (a.k.a. "cheat sheets") at home. However, in class they tend to become a distraction, and can lead to an over-intellectualization of the practice. Worse, they reduce this wonderful practice to a mere scavenger-hunt of poses to complete.

Just know that hundreds of thousands of people have learned Ashtanga Vinyasa. You can learn it, too, and sooner than you think. So have faith and enthusiasm. In a Mysore class, you can draw strength, support and comfort from the community of people practicing around you. Know that everyone — including me — has learned the sequence, addressed uncertainty, and faced not knowing, just as you might be.

How Often Should I Practice?

The practice room is open between 6:00 and 9:00 a.m. Monday–Friday. The Ashtanga method is intended to be a daily practice, and students are encouraged to make a commitment to practice at least three times a week for a month at a time.

Traditionally, we practice every day except for Saturdays and moon days.

It may be very difficult at first to commit to a daily practice, and it often takes time to establish this. Regular attendance is encouraged, although a few times a week combined with a self-practice at home is sufficient.

Drop-ins are fine for out-of-town visitors or others with an established practice.

What Time Can I Arrive?

Doors open at 6 a.m. You can arrive at any point until class ends at 9 a.m. If the door is locked, stand on the sidewalk and press the button until I come out and let you in. I'd prefer everyone start by 8, but if you have to choose between arriving at 8:30 or no practice, show up at 8:30.

Do I Have to Get Up That Early?

Listen buttercup, it's time to rip off the Band-Aid. To develop a Mysore practice is to deepen, broaden and evolve your own Yoga practice. You'll also support and be supported by a community of like-minded people.

Some morning Mysore practices are like stepping into a jet stream — you are borne along on a vital circuit of energy that is greater than you, more ordinary than you, and nothing but you, all at once. When you are finished, you will lie down and take rest, and you will rise from your rest like Lazarus to find the world profoundly changed and yet exactly the same.

For that to happen, you have to get up in the morning.

Despite what your mom told you, you are not a unique snowflake. You are a diurnal mammal, which means you function best during sunlight.

You are not a "night person."

"I don't do mornings" or "I'm not a morning person" are excuses.

Put your alarm clock across the room. When it rings, get up.

What If I'm Not Flexible in the Morning?

To paraphrase a quote I once saw at Vancouver Ashtanga, you're never too dirty to take a shower. If you wait until you're flexible enough in order to take a Yoga class, you will wait until death. On a purely physical level, consistent morning stretching eventually allows you to perform movements that require considerable flexibility with little or no warm-up.

Do I Have to Go to Work All Sweaty?

The delightful environs of Yoga Pearl also include luxurious showers, organic soap, and a towel service. Yoga Pearl also houses Prasad Cafe, which features raw cheesecake, Bachelor bars, gluten-free cookies, and other breakfast items.

What Should I Wear?

Wear loose, comfortable clothing in which you can sweat. Socks (and mittens) will not work. You are not obligated to wear spandex, Speedos, or Lululemon's latest.

Should I Eat Before Class?

As a rough rule of thumb, try not to eat or drink anything 2 hours before practicing. Over time, you'll figure out what and how to best serve your unique nutrition needs.

What About Hygiene?

Please try to wear clean clothes and shower before class. Deodorants and scented oils are okay, just don't bathe in them. If you have to ask if you're wearing too much, then you're wearing too much. Don't slather on the Tiger Balm and Ben-Gay. They won't help much anyway. Gentlemen, if you wear Axe, then beware the Axe Effect.

MYSORE GUILT

We last returned to Mysore, India, in fall 2005. It's strange to type that date because it seems and feels so long ago! As a family we've chosen to pursue other interests, among them more frequent trips to visit Tim Miller in Encinitas.

Still, this decision isn't a negation of the place. It's true, though, that my relationship to Mysore is a complex one. While I've chosen more frequent trips to Encinitas, I do from time to time feel a small but noticeable drive to return to India.

My initial trip there was sparked in part by my first meeting with Pattabhi Jois in New York City during one of his annual world tours. I had such a terrific time practicing in the Puck Building that I began to organize my life to spend an uncertain amount of time in India. Subsequently I sold, gave away, or threw out all my belongings, quit my job, and abandoned my car in order to visit Mysore.

Unfortunately, at Pattabhi Jois' age, and given the vast numbers of students then in Mysore, I didn't have the opportunity to develop a personal relationship with him. He vaguely recognized me as Tim's student and perhaps thought my tattoos were humorous. The asana experience there was, to put it mildly, very powerful. Still, though, since he passed in 2009, that gravitic pull to Mysore has noticeably lessened.

When I began practicing in Encinitas, a trip to Mysore was a discrete yet frequent conversational current. Meaning there was no expectation or pressure to travel there, but "When are you going to Mysore?" was a common refrain. The feel in Encinitas has, of course, changed somewhat during the last several years.

The Ashtanga Vinyasa community in Portland doesn't really have that vague cloud of social pressure to travel to Mysore, quite simply because it's not a topic. I expect I may inadvertently encourage people to travel to India, though, when I share India stories or pass along the aspects of this practice that I picked up in Mysore.

Still, although the urge to return may have lessened, it still occurs and is only sharpened by the fact that I'm not Authorized by the Ashtanga Yoga Institute. I'm sure this urge flowers in part from small seeds of nagging doubts about my own validity and legitimacy as a teacher.

Official recognition is a tricky beast, isn't it? "Official" approval and recognition by the leading Ashtanga Vinyasa institution, the holders of this lineage and tradition, would paper over any of my personal shortcomings or doubts. I could really lean on that recognition, too; if people asked why I suggest certain postures or sequences, I could then say, "Because that's how they do it in Mysore."

I also have the tendency to "collect," and for me the pursuit of recognition becomes a goal unto itself, a thing pursued for no other reason than to collect it. The "Collector" mentality gives the illusion of direction and meaning, and yet is another elaborate method of avoidance or disengagement with life as it is now. In other words, getting Authorized, or even Certified — well, it's something to do, right?

I also get the itch to visit Mysore because the Ashtanga Vinyasa community is so spread out that it's the only place to catch up with old friends, as well as Sharath, and meet new members of the growing community. While Ashtanga Vinyasa is a solitary practice — only you can do it — in a Mysore setting, it's not practiced in solitude. I found a vast connection to like-minded and interesting people there, and that was a good thing.

Guruji's tours were such a great opportunity for everyone to come together in one place and for one reason. Even if they were in an air-conditioned gymnasium, they were so very powerful.

The in-breath brings a great many people into your life, and of course the out-breath takes them away again. They come, they go. For me, part of the Yoga practice is to acknowledge and work with the current situation of my life. Not as I wish it to be one day in Mysore, and not as it was the last time I was in Mysore, but as it is today, right now.

So a journey to Mysore could be a flight from my life. It could even be a path towards so-called self-validation. But then it could also be a holiday or a pilgrimage. I know I'll return to Mysore some day, and I look forward to it. I realize now, though, that I don't need to be there to honor this tradition.

I do that every time I practice..

MY SIDDHIS

I've compiled a list of all the siddhis I have developed as a result of years of daily practice.

For those of you unfamiliar with yogic terminology, "siddhis" here refers to the paranormal powers available to very advanced yogis such as myself. For example, the venerable Indian guru Sai Baba can materialize vibhuti, or holy ash, as well as various faux-gold trinkets such as pens and pocket watches. He can also make disappear inquiries into his relations with underage boys.

While I'm not quite that advanced, here are some of my abilities.

Radio Station Presets

When I rent a car, the radio station will come preset to the best radio stations that area has to offer, no matter which area I am in! Remember, I do not ask for these gifts. They simply manifest.

Parking Spot Ability

The rest of you circle the 17th and Valencia block in San Francisco perhaps 10 or 15 times as you look for a parking spot. Me? Two times, tops.

Supermarket Discount
While most people have to sign up to get supermarket rewards and club cards, this discount mysteriously manifests itself for me, unasked, at the time I check out.

Lint and Cat-hair Repellant
Despite now having two cats, my hip black clothing radiates a magnetic charge that repels their hair, as well as lint.

Movie Theater Preview Avoidance
No matter what time I leave the house, I enter the movie theater seconds before the main feature begins. I am an eminently desirable companion on any movie-going experience.

Book Absorption
When I read a book, you can speak, shout or scream at me — in fact, my wife has often attempted to speak directly into my ear-hole from millimeters away — and I will not even know you are there! It's not that I ignore you. It's just that, as my gift operates, you do not exist.

Saving Throw +20 Against Breath Weapons
I am well nigh undefeatable when I face dragons, gorgons, or other magical breath-weapon-based creatures.

Party Invisibility
When it's time to leave a party or social gathering, usually at the 20-minute mark, I have the uncanny ability to find and use the nearest exit without saying goodbye to a single person!

A LETTER TO THE EDITOR OF *YOGA JOURNAL*

Dear Madam,

I sincerely laud your endeavors at *Yoga Journal*.
The editorial direction and the pictorial content that you and your shareholders have determined to be the most lucrative — that which will attract advertising dollars aimed at 30-to-40-year-old middle- and upper-middle-class Caucasian women — has indeed attracted top-tier women's Yoga clothing brands.

However, as a testosterone-laden, red-blooded heterosexual male (can you say householder? Cha-ching!), I must also congratulate you on so successfully capturing another important Yoga demographic and, like true market innovators, meeting a heretofore-unknown demand. While *Namarupa* remains the premier magazine for Yoga-related philosophy, discourse, photography, and interviews, you remain the only high-quality glossy Yoga jerk-off mag on the market.

Kudos!

Sincerely,
Et cetera, et cetera.

P.S. I anxiously await your "Girls of the *Bhagavad Gita*" pictorial. "Hardtail," indeed!

AGE 19

I was a young man with a restless, rootless, unscratchable itch. Apartments, cities, states, countries, jobs, careers — I was blown among and between them by unseen winds, no port a home and no destination final.

My dad worked first for Ford Aerospace and then the U.S. State Department, and beginning at about 9 months of age, my family moved from country to country, state to state, roughly every other year of my entire life. You could say that extreme cultural, social and personal transience was the norm.

So it was a big deal to me when, at age 19, I put all of my belongings in the back of a silver and rust four-door 1980 Honda Civic and caravanned to California. Although it was only the latest of many relocations in my life, it was the first I'd ever undertaken at my own initiative and to a place of my own choosing.

By "belongings," I mean two crates of books, a duffel bag, and a gigantic albatross of a TV that took up the entire backseat. I followed my friend Tom's maroon '88 Ford Shitbox 2,300 miles from Milwaukee, Wisconsin, to Encinitas, California. It was a marathon 2-and-a-half day drive fueled by quarts of coffee, fistfuls of No-Doz, and 2-liter bottles of Mountain Dew. There was a pre-dawn stretch through Utah characterized by frightening and vivid hallucinations, as painted freeway lines floated off the pavement and giant hairy bat-shapes flapped their wings just beyond the headlights' reach.

When we crossed the Nevada border, I was eating No-Doz every few minutes like M&Ms and trying to pee into empty 2-liters. I was left with maddening phantom total-body itches and piss-stained shorts.

Tom had gone to high school with a kid named Marc, and Marc's parents had moved to Encinitas some years before. We landed at their house, and then the three of us rented an apartment in a synthetic, manicured apartment complex in Cardiff, just a few minutes drive down the coast from Encinitas. The postcards called it "Cardiff-by-the-Sea."

Tom returned to Milwaukee after a few short months while I soldiered on. After 2 years in the apartment complex, Marc and I opted to relocate to new digs. We were also served an eviction notice. We settled in Encinitas proper, in a complex of ramshackle beach cottages on the corner of Third and A Streets.

Rent for the two bedroom was $675 a month. I paid $325 for my own room while Marc and another housemate split the rest. The cottage had no insulation; moisture beaded the concrete walls and anything in the closets grew mold. The wooden steps off the side porch were rotted, and we later discovered there was no plumbing connected to the shower drain — the water dumped right into the ground under the house.

Still, we could see the sand volleyball courts on Moonlight Beach from our front lawn, and we would bomb steep and gravelly Third Street on our skateboards on the way to Manhattan Giant Pizza, where foot-long cheese slices were $1, tax included. A slice for breakfast, lunch, and dinner meant my daily food budget was often $3. It was a young and poor bachelor's paradise. Of course, the beach cottages were eventually torn down and there are condos there now.

I moved for brief stints to Venice Beach and Hollywood before landing once again in Encinitas, now just three blocks down from the ramshackle beach cottages, on the corner of Fourth and D Streets.

From Encinitas, I relocated to downtown San Diego and then to San Francisco before returning, once more, to Encinitas — and once again to Fourth and D Street. This time I was in a different apartment, yet in the exact same complex in which I had lived years before.

I remember the date I returned from San Francisco to Encinitas — October 5, 2001 — because it was the first monthly check I wrote to the Ashtanga Yoga Center.

The point of all this downtown Encinitas geography is that somehow, during the endless and seemingly arbitrary peregrinations of my late teens and twenties, Ashtanga Vinyasa Yoga appeared in my life — and then continued to appear, as for 5 years I lived within sight of the Ashtanga Yoga Center on E Street. In fact, I seemed to orbit it, as despite moving to four different cities, each time I'd return to a location just a few blocks away. I would walk past the place several times a day, and almost always three nights a week on my way to The Saloon, the local bar, which was around the corner.

I've long since gotten rid of the giant TV and the rusted 1980 Civic. I no longer live in what I remember as bachelor pads but were in reality hovels. I don't cringe when my food budget exceeds $3 a day. From time to time I still get a fierce, burning wanderlust, but overall I'm very much more settled.

It's easy, now, to look back on this process as inevitable. It's easy to shape it into one seamless narrative. But in truth, the appearance and reappearance of Ashtanga Vinyasa Yoga was and remains the result of a moment-by-moment weaving of choices, both large and small.

EXPRESSWAY TO FLEXIBILITY

Here are several speedy and sure-fire ways to insure flexibility, beyond the ol' "consistent practice" cliché. Bor-ing! Clearly the sooner you can fit your leg behind your head, the sooner life will get a lot easier.

Dysentery
Spend five or six days bed-ridden, pant-legs tied off around your ankles to prevent the torrent of shit from running onto the bed, chair and floor, and subsisting on crackers and soda water. You'll come back to your mat super bendy and pliable. Oh, and for those of you looking for a magic weight-loss plan, look no further than dysentery. Your body will literally eat the fat and muscle right off your bones.

Food Poisoning
Not only will a bout of food poisoning render you as limber as a contortionist, you'll also develop an intense bhakti practice, too. You will never chant, pray, or more wholeheartedly dedicate your existence to a higher power as fervently as when you have no control over your bowels.

Cip-Zoxx

I asked the chemists in Gokulam, a neighborhood in Mysore, what medicine they had for back pain. They sold me a sheaf of horse-pills called Cip-Zoxx. One part ibuprofen, one part acetaminophen, and one part melty-face. The third magic ingredient is a wicked muscle relaxer. You'll feel your vertebrae moving out of place during kapotasana and you won't care.

Sleeplessness

Your Yoga practice after a sleepless three-day bender in Las Vegas is, shall we say, loosey-goosey.

Crystal Methamphetamine

I have no personal experience with crystal meth, but when I lived in San Francisco I used to practice next to a guy who wore double-extra baggy raver jeans. He had jaundice-yellow sweat-stains on the neck and armpits of his shirt, and he emitted the tangy smell of ether as well as the crunching sound of grinding teeth. He told me he practiced two or three times a day, and that crystal meth really helped him "get into that groove."

YOU KNOW IT AIN'T EASY

Sometimes it's a tightrope act. I want to practice every day, as teachers and texts prescribe, and because, y'know, it's what feels good. So I shuffle and organize my life in whatever ways are appropriate to make that happen. I negotiate with employers, clients, my wife and my daughter in order to carve out the requisite time.

One side of the tightrope is no practice at all. However, an established practice has its own pitfalls. Once the time is marked out, the space for the practice set, and the morning ritual established — get up, wash face, pranayama for 45 minutes, sit for 20, chug espresso, drive to Yoga studio, unroll mat — the entire thing becomes what I've worked so hard to build. That is, routine. With all the negative connotations that word implies, such as rote, habitual and unconscious.

It never gets easier, either. My wife's body in the pre-dawn hour has not gotten less warm, less comforting, less inviting, and the thought of turning off the alarm has not become less tempting. This practice stubbornly refuses to do itself. I still have to start it, tend it like a banked fire, and expend however skillfully the energy required to complete it.

My wife and I both keep practicing, though, supporting each other as best we can, reaching to the texts, ancient and new, for impetus and inspiration, and modeling the long-time practitioner with whom we studied for those many years, the man we call our teacher.

A practice is like sailing a ship, a lifelong journey during which we make minute and constant adjustments of our course in the face of unexpected gale winds, long periods of daily routine, and patches of becalmed sea.

SHANKARA AND BANDHAS

Here's a little more of the philosophy that girds the practice of Ashtanga Vinyasa as taught by Pattabhi Jois. Jois (or Guruji!) was of the Hoysala Brahmin caste, a subset of the immensely popular Smarta Brahmins whose root teacher or sadguru is Adi Shankaracharya.

Shankaracharya, who most likely lived in the Eighth Century C.E., was one of the giants of Indian philosophy and arguably the forefather of Advaita Vedanta. Much of Shankaracharya's work is available online; there are also many later Tantric texts that bear his name that were not written by him.

His *Aparokshanubhuti* is online and worth a read on your moon day, especially as it addresses many techniques and practices we cultivate in Ashtanga Vinyasa, among them mula bandha.

As lines 114 and 115 read:

> 114. That which is the root of all existence and on which the restraint of the mind is based is called the restraining root [mulabandha] which should always be adopted since it is fit for raja-yogins.

115. Absorption in the uniform Reality should be known as the equipoise of the limbs [dehasamya]. Otherwise, mere straightening of the body like that of a dried-up tree is no equipoise.

The practice of mula bandha is fit for a King! Also doubtless fit for the Queen of Kings (or Rajarajeshwari). You can get an idea of the tenets of Advaita Vedanta by reading the text, which is available online.

WHAT FIRST SERIES TAUGHT ME

I came to the Primary Series when I was 23. I was stiff, weak, and suffering profoundly from the disconnect between my intellect and my physical and emotional intelligence. My consciousness orbited about 6 inches above and just to the rear of my skull.

The Primary Series, "Yoga Chikitsa" as it's known in Sanskrit, or "Yoga therapy," definitely fulfilled a therapeutic function for me. In my first Yoga class, a sense of awareness spread through my skin, bones, muscle, and sinew in a way that was a total surprise and yet entirely inevitable.

After the peregrinations of my early 20s, when I lived in San Diego, Los Angeles and San Francisco, I once again settled in Encinitas and began practicing six days a week. I had a flexible job that allowed me to drift in to the office between 9:15 and

9:30 a.m., and so I began attending Mysore classes at Tim Miller's Ashtanga Yoga Center.[2]

The series taught me strength, both physical and mental. It showed me that discipline was a skill that improved with practice. I began to pay attention to what I put in my body because that which sustained me directly influenced how I moved, felt, and thought. I began to more consciously organize my life and the direction of my attention to sustain an early-morning practice. In general, this meant an earlier bedtime and less partying.

On a wonderfully mundane level, the forward bending and hip mobility in the Primary Series were so immediate and intense that I simply had to learn vinyasa or else I would have died.

Pattabhi Jois used to say, "Primary Series, very important!" Yoga Chikitsa was the way I learned and practiced absorption, dissolution, and direct participation that is the wonderful byproduct of engaging ujjayi breathing, vinyasa, drishti and the bandhas. Yoga Chikitsa is how I learned to practice both the diffusion and collection of effort, attention, and breathing, which is what I understand to be prana.

There's also something wonderfully communal about Primary Series. Every Friday around the world, rooms full of people inhale and exhale, rise and fold, as one.

I don't know specifically where my consciousness, my heart-and-mind, now resides, but it doesn't seem as disconnected as it once was. That is a good thing. I credit the Primary Series. Sometimes it's easy, sometimes it's inexplicably difficult. But it's always there for the practicing.

---

2 At that time I don't believe Tim taught the Primary Series in the Mysore style, which is pose-by-pose. At least, he never taught it to me that way. So it was during Tuesday's 7 a.m. led Primary Series class, in which Tim unrolled his mat to lead the class, and said nothing but the pose name and "Five," to indicate the end of the pose, that I eventually learned the Primary Series in its entirety.

HIMSA

I copped a pair of used Chuck Taylors (blue) at Buffalo Exchange. They were $14.99 and, as the tag said, "gently worn."

This morning some douchebag stole 'em from the front of the Yoga studio. Never mind the logistics — like, who's trolling around at 8 a.m. on the second floor of an empty building? Who would steal a pair of wet, dirty, well-fucking-worn pair of Chuck Taylors?

After the incredulity of the situation passed — yes, my shoes were really gone — I gleefully entertained fantasies of laying hands on this individual, this shoe-thief, catching him in the act, as it were, and administering frontier justice to him, a stiff dose of pure himsa, "harm" or "wounding."

Also, I gleefully entertained a little bit of himsa for anyone who might chirp, "Guess it's just another lesson in non-attachment!" Not so much for the sentiment, of course, but for refusing to acknowledge the dynamic, energizing reality of anger. Anger exists. It's not going away, nor would we want it to. Classical Hindu ethics consider anger (krodha) one of the "Six Poisons" (shad vargas or doshas) around the heart, to be "purified."

Yet they also make space for Krodha Bhairava, a form of Shiva (one of many) as elemental rage, as well as the rasa (or "taste") raudra, or fury.

All this meaning, anger, rage and fury can be poison encircling your heart — but this poison (or taste, your choice) exists and must be addressed.

My shoe-theft anger sparked, swelled, then faded. I enjoyed and was entertained by the fantasies that unspooled in my head. I commiserated with the wife and have since funneled the heat of that anger into this post, which has served as a lightning rod to ground and channel it.

Of course, now I'm in the market for another affordable pair of Chucks. I'll take 'em "gently used," too.

IMBALANCES

Asana practice lends itself to different lenses of varying depths and utility. It's easy to get trapped on the materialist and reductionist side of the map, a place where asanas are mere assemblages of body parts.

Consequently, our personal list of physical injuries, tendencies, and idiosyncrasies become problems to be solved or obstacles to be overcome through Yoga. This view reduces Yoga asana to physical therapy.

The subtler thinking that accompanies this reduction is the deep cherishment of these idiosyncrasies and injuries, and their acceptance as limiting beliefs.

A.G. Mohan writes that Krishnamacharya, Pattabhi Jois' teacher, had a useful multi-level framework to view asana practice: as spiritual practice (upasana), therapy (chikitsa), and fitness (shiksa).

So this means we're not shallow for our curiosity about anatomy and physical expression, as though we're somehow less "serious" for not seeing Yoga asana practice only in "spiritual" terms. I believe an intense focus and interest in asana mechanics and anatomy is a stage through which we must pass.

Also, it's useful to observe that Patanjali suggests that attention to our body (sauca) is essential, and that sickness (vyadhi) is an obstacle. The *Taittriya Upanishad*, which Guruji loved to quote, suggests that our food-body (anna maya kosha) is the first of five nested shells or sheaths (panchakoshas). Both Patanjali and the Panchakosha map of our experience suggest that our bodies are vital, important, and inextricably related with other, subtler levels and layers.

Still, while I don't believe one needs to be an anatomist to teach asana, it can still enrich one's practice to pay attention to the physical food-body realm. Just don't get stuck there!

I've been fortunate to hold space for Mysore-style classes since 2004, and most of the gift of that time has been quite simply to watch and observe hundreds (thousands?) of bodies as they move through the same ritualized sequence of interlinked postures.

In that time I've come to observe a couple common tendencies, whether in people off the street/couch, athletes, dancers or performers, or long-time yoginis.

These are broad generalizations, of course, and don't apply to all equally.

Also, I have chosen to ignore medical terminology.

1. SHOULDER IMBALANCE; FRONT/BACK

Humans are an anterior and front-facing species.

So it's pretty much inevitable that the muscles on the front of our body are stronger than the muscles on the back, especially on our grabby bits.

We push and pull with our chest and the front and sides of our arms.

So generally, this means our upper back, as well as the backs of the shoulders and arms, are a bit weaker.

There is the belief that Ashtanga Vinyasa people have hurt shoulders. Given the high repetitions of chaturangas, lolasanas, uth pluthis, jump-backs and urdvha dhanurasanas, this is definitely a shadow element of which we ought to be aware.

Generally when a person tells me they have shoulder pain, I watch them lower into chaturanga and, nine times out of 10, the top of their arm bone rolls forward in their shoulder — the muscles that support the wing-bone and the backs of the shoulder are unable to keep the arm centered in its socket.

This imbalance is also why, for example, your hands slide together in pinche mayurasana, or you have a hard time keeping the elbows in when pushing up into urdvha dhanurasana.

2. LEG IMBALANCE; INNER/OUTER

If we all squatted a lot this wouldn't be an issue. This generally is not an issue in former ballerinas or martial artists; that is, people who have done a lot of kicking and leg swings.

This is why you have to pay conscious attention to make sure your knee tracks your toes during virabadrasana. Usually I see the knee waggle inward and the foot flatten.

3. SHORT HIP FLEXORS

Generally, we sit a lot, so the front of our hips shorten and the backs of our legs get weak.

We do no hip extension in the Primary Series until backbends, so this one's harder to untangle, though tiraing mukkha eka pada paschimattanasana is sometimes a good clue.

WHAT TO DO ABOUT IT

I didn't want to present a problem and then not offer a solution; however, I wrote five pages of postural suggestions that, upon re-reading, caused my own eyes to dry up and fall out of my skull from boredom.

So there're a lot of great technical manuals out there: Maehle's book, if for nothing but the technical info. Swenson's book is also great because it's simple.

The act of writing out the alignment suggestions was therapeutic for me, though, because look, let's face it: you just have to show up consistently and practice the Primary Series with a teacher/friend who has a good eye for energy lines — or at the very least, has practiced for a little while themselves and can tell when something may hurt further down the line.

To get too worried about correcting structural imbalances and we drift into the realm of physical therapy. We strip Ashtanga of its inherent power and become mired in the problem/solution dialectic.

I think this can be okay for a period of time because it can also reveal a lot about our expectations of a Yoga practice: Do we expect it to take us from one state to another, one totally unlike the one before? Do we consider life a problem to be solved? Are we inherently broken and in need of fixing?

These feel like more important questions to savor.

YOGA ROUTINE, ENCINITAS 2002

I have two alarms rigged up, my cell phone and an alarm clock. The cell phone is on the table by my bed, and it goes off first. I turn it off. A few minutes later, my radio-alarm clock goes off. It's positioned across the room on my bookshelf.

When I lived in San Francisco I practiced at Ahimsa Yoga, a studio run by Alice Joanou. After a few months of three-to-four-times-a-week led classes, I felt that there was more to this Yoga, and that I just wasn't going "deep" enough.

I asked Alice what the next level was. She informed me that traditionally Ashtanga Yoga is practiced in the Mysore style, which means a set, predetermined sequence practiced in a self-paced class setting six days a week, at 6 or 7 in the morning.

I was floored. "*Six* days a week? At 6 in the morning? Are you out of your fucking mind? There is no way I could get out bed that early! Do you know how stiff I am in the morning? No *way*."

Alice told me that she was the same way, until she got a tip on how to get up early. It proved to be some of the wisest advice

I've ever received: put your alarm clock on the far side of the room so you have to stand up to shut it off.[3]

It works. Nowadays the alarm fires at 4:30. Generally I smash the snooze bar and drift for another 10 minutes. I've also set my radio alarm clock to a country-western station, which pulls me out of bed right quick.

I shower, more to rinse off the sleep than get clean. I will shortly be leaking sweat anyway. I turn on the computer and fire up the brand-new espresso machine I bought at Target.

From 5 to about 6 I answer and send emails for work and/or read. I leave for the studio at about five 'til 6. The studio is literally two blocks. I drive because I leave for work immediately after practice. The last few days it's been dark when I've left the house, and the weather has been cold as hell.

I don't know if my experience of and with Yoga is now "deeper." It doesn't seem to matter. This practice is like a loose thread, or a sore tooth. I can't help but pick at it.

---

[3] She also gave me two great tips on teaching Yoga: "Don't bang your students," and "Fart in class every once in a while."

FLENSING

Sometimes I do things because I think I *should* do them, rather than because I actually enjoy and derive sustenance from them.

I always felt obligated to read Daniel Pinchbeck. I labored through his books *Breaking Open the Head* and *2012,* and I even attended a speaking appearance he made at Powell's Books here in Portland. He seemed to be engaged in ways of thinking and looking at the world that mirrored my own. After all, he's interested in "breaking open the head," and isn't the practice of Yoga really just the same thing?

It turns out it's not, and today I came to the realization I was following Pinchbeck's blogs and reading his books out of a sense of obligation rather than interest. So I axed my sub to his blog as well as the other site he curates, Reality Sandwich.

Pinchbeck seemed like he had some interesting things to say, and Reality Sandwich seemed like it would provide insightful, thought-provoking and inspirational stories about tapping into a deeper, more profound sense of sacredness and intimacy. They'd even publish Yoga-related stories or posts, through which I'd dutifully slog.

I came to the realization that Reality Sandwich and Pinchbeck's books were just drug stories and chemical tourism.

Let's not kid ourselves. You can't get "it" by drinking ayahuasca. The implication is that the reality accessed through ayahuasca is somehow separate and other from your everyday reality. Unfortunately, your everyday reality is the one to which you will always and forevermore return when the high wears off.

What's more, there is no way to affirm or deny with any certainty that there are tribes of hyper-dimensional machine-elves attempting to communicate with us via DMT and "spirit molecules."

If you buy into these stories, congratulations. You now require DMT or ayahuasca, chemical sacraments administered by priests or drug dealers, to act as an intermediary. At best you've further externalized Source and reinforced a sense of separateness between sacredness and yourself. At worst you've just deified another omnipotent supernatural figure, the "machine elves," who now require their own sacrament, DMT.

When I was younger, psychenauts like Daniel Pinchbeck, Timothy Leary and Terence McKenna seemed cool. But back then, I was more occupied with chemically stretching the confines of my own consciousness. Maybe I've mellowed as I've aged, or maybe I just stretched things as far as they needed to be stretched. I can't help but feel that any state of consciousness that refuses to stay "stretched" without some substance — and in fact, any substance that subsequently causes deep depression or anxiety — is worthless, and nothing more than a temporary state. It's one I can choose to enjoy, or not, but regardless it's a state that will inevitably end.

You want to get wasted? Then get wasted. Don't get me wrong, I am not a tee-totaler or a straight-edger. I'm all for getting wasted, and in fact spent several years of my life doing so in various ways. It was mind-expanding, for sure, and there are times when perhaps the radical reduction or expansion of consciousness is called for.

This dovetails with my general lack of use for mystic union. It's great when it arises, and I'm not saying we need to run Rumi out of town, because mystics can tell us a lot about the outer shores of consciousness. I see a lot of big problems, though, when those fringes become enshrined as goals or end-states to be chased or attained. I believe they call those people "bliss bunnies."

What's that bullshit book fobbed on every aspiring Yoga student, the Paramahamsa Yogananda one? The one you can find a dozen copies of at any book swap in India? *Autobiography of a Yogi*? It's filled with tons of instances of mystic rapture so great, so deep, that Paramahamsa couldn't speak, feed himself or, one would imagine, wipe his ass.

That pretty much covers a broad range of books, by the way. The field of pop Yoga literature is filled with books by guys describing bouts of mystic rapture and union, guys like Sai Baba and the Krishnamurthis, J. and U.G., the crabby one.

Along those lines, I've just finished a book on Papaji that I found at the local Goodwill. Papaji's the guy behind Gangaji and Eli Jaxon Bear, and he has some interesting things to say about the state of non-dual consciousness or awakening. What does he say as for how he "achieved" it? Not much. His description of states of bliss sound a lot like the chillout/nitrous room on day two of a three-day rave: rapturous, wide-eyed, drooling, insensate.

So what good is bliss? This is the Twenty-first Century, after all. A click of the mouse and I can get peyote, mescaline, MDMA, ibogaine, DMT, ayahuasca. All that bliss is available on the Internets.

In addition to the inevitable hangovers the bliss powders provide — my favorite is the "chucha," or ayahuasca's explosive projectile "sacred diarrhea" — I'm ambivalent about people glorifying some great, bliss-filled ecstatic condition, if only because life contains so much more than that.

Life is great and wondrous, sure, but man, it's shitty, too, and people can be mean and small-minded — try "taking" someone's "spot" at the Shala in Mysore — and there's sadness, and despair, and all that. Most of the time life is just ordinary. Terrifyingly, achingly ordinary. You get to wait in line at the DMV, you get to clean up cat barf off the rug, you get to hang out on hold when you call your cable company. All this ordinary bullshit is the package, too. It is not separate from all the wonder and awe, it's not separate from the suffering and pain.

So back to Pinchbeck: I don't know how sustained use of ayahuasca will help with anything more than momentary flashes of mystic union, which, if we take a moment to use the Ashtanga Yoga structure, is but one of the eight limbs, samadhi.

I know Patanjali suggests that ausadhi, or "herbs," can be one of the tools to use to remove the veils. But he also lists "vyadhi," or sickness, as the first obstacle to practice. If you're using herbs that make you sick, your herbs are no good, and if your herbs cause any of the subsequent barriers to practice — doubt, "stuck"ness, langour, etc., etc. — then the herbs or powders are not working, are they?

I've come to understand that I practice Yoga not to suppress or eliminate the good, the bad, and the ordinary, but to recognize them for what they are — momentary thoughts, emotions and evaluations that arise and pass away, to be savored as such.

Some yearned-for "return" to an Edenic Golden Age, one filled with machine-elves, Mother Earth worship, or the aliens who make crop circles, is to attempt, through sheer force of will, to turn the Universe into what we desire or hope it to be.

WHAT I KNOW ABOUT YOGA AND FOOD

The Ashtanga Vinyasa Yoga practice being what it is — daily, consistent, fixed — I naturally began to track correlations between my eating habits and my Yoga practice. As a result, I've experimented with different eating habits, regimens or philosophies.

A few of the systems I've encountered and/or tried directly myself include Paleo (no grains, legumes or dairy), vegetarianism, veganism, macrobiotics, raw foodism, fruitarianism, scavengism, breatharianism (or, as an old teacher of mine called it, "male anorexia") and uropathy, the drinking of one's own urine.

A woman once asked Pattabhi Jois if dark chocolate would make her more flexible. Guruji responded with a vigorous "Yes!" Milk chocolate, with its milk and sugar, is apparently a very sattvic food. Guruji, I should add, had a legendary sweet tooth. So the next several mornings, before 5 a.m. class, the woman hurriedly gobbled down bits of dark chocolate in front of the shala gates.

I don't know if the chocolate made her more flexible. Still, if you can work out a way to have the consumption of chocolate legitimized and endorsed as part of your Yoga practice, I say go for it.

Unfortunately and in all honesty, at this point I can't say with any certainty that eating certain kinds of food specifically effects in any way my experience on the Yoga mat. Meat, no meat; raw, cooked. Still, I can make a very few broad generalizations based on my experience.

Drink a Lot of Water
I don't exactly measure it out, but I try to get at least 64 ounces a day. The tapas of a daily practice refined my discrimination to the point where I realized I often ate when I was thirsty. I misinterpreted my body's signals, and therefore walked around perpetually dehydrated.

Begin a Daily Practice
This is seemingly unrelated to the food you're eating. But in my experience, the daily or near-daily practice of the Primary Series of Ashtanga Yoga sensitized me to what I was putting into and moving out of my body. Just as importantly it also sensitized me to what was *not* moving out of my body.

Basically, what it emphasized to me was my relationship to my food and digestive process, as well as my mental, physical and spiritual states relating to food.

Bigger Lunch, Smaller Dinner
When I stayed out late with the work crew for an extended happy hour, and horked down margaritas as well as baskets of free garlic bread and a mega-dinner of spinach and garlic raviolis, the next morning I felt a tad sluggish.

When I undereat, though, I feel bendy and light for a day or so, which then degenerates into floppiness, weakness, and light-headedness.

I'm interested to learn how anorexic and bulimics Ashtangis manage to pull it off. I imagine the physiological checks they write on their bodies get cashed that much sooner due to the demands of the Ashtanga practice.

Lots of Good Sleep

The less sleep, the more flexible and strong. This, though, is a very slippery slope. I've had brilliant practices after two hours of sleep, but this is simply not sustainable on a day-to-day basis. We also do our most important recovery while we sleep, too, both physical, mental and emotional. So I can't understate the importance of sleep. By "sleep," I mean 7 to 9 hours in a pitch-black room. That's right, 7 to 9 hours.

SUBMIT TO PRACTICE

New York Times douchebag Stanley Fish reviewed Matthew Crawford's book *Shop Class as Soulcraft: An Inquiry into the Value of Work*.[4]

I was immediately struck by the application of Crawford's thinking to an established, systemic Yoga practice. As Fish writes:

> Crawford associates ... 'remote control' knowledge with liberalism, a way of thinking that has at its center the individual self unburdened 'by attachments to others and radically free,' a self whose chief commitment and obligation is to its own 'creativity.'

Fish continues:

> "Crawford prefers to the ethic of individual creativity and its 'rhetoric of freedom' the ethic of submission to facts 'that do not arise from the human will.' It is that submission, he says, that characterizes the work of craftsmen, artisans and musicians. 'One can't be a musician without ... subjecting one's fingers to the discipline of frets or keys.'

---

4 *New York Times,* "Think Again," June 14, 2009.

> Whereas craftsmanship 'means dwelling on a task for a long time and going deeply into it,' the 'preferred role model' of the radically free liberal self 'is the management consultant, who swoops in and out and whose very pride lies in his lack of particular expertise.'"

Here Crawford might as well be discussing the difference between buffet-style and systemic Yoga practices. Buffet-style Yoga is an extension of the self and beholden only to its practitioners' "creativity."

A systematic approach to Yoga has an established sequence of asanas, pranayamas and seated techniques that cannot "arise from the human will." I am reminded of Krishna's famous definition of Yoga, in the *Bhagavad Gita*, as "skill in action," the residue of which, Yoga, arises only after "dwelling on a task for a long time and going deeply into it."

Here we can also default to Pattabhi Jois' simpler, famous four-word dictum: "Practice, practice. Long time."

Then there's also the idea of "submission." It is a great paradox that freedom, liberation, or moksha, or even relationship, arises only after submitting to a discipline and rigor beyond the scope of "human will." To describe this paradox, Richard Freeman uses the image of the ouroboros, the alchemical symbol of the snake swallowing its own tail.

A practice like Ashtanga Vinyasa is, by its very nature, the limiting or closing off of potentiality, of choice, of freedom. Yet it is only by rubbing against the edges of the practice — these poses, in this order, using these techniques — that freedom arises.

RAMESH BALSEKAR IN MUMBAI

The taxi ride from our hotel, near Bombay Hospital, to Ramesh's flat on Gamadia Road costs 40 Rupees. It's hard to tell if that means it's near or far 'cause prices in Mumbai are hyper-jacked. We find the building easily because we follow a bronzed-tan Westerner wearing an Om T-shirt.

We barge into the living room about 5 minutes after Ramesh's talk has begun. He holds them every morning from 9 to 10:30, and today, a Saturday, there are perhaps 30 people gathered, mostly Westerners, in the spacious but plain living room. Tara, Rowan and I sit in a swing-couch at one end of the room. The windows are open, so we get a nice breeze, and it's still too early for the sweltering Mumbai heat to render all movement, all thought, and all speech superfluous at best and impossible at worst. On the wall are several portraits of Ramana Maharshi and one of Nisargdaj Maharaj. Among them is a portrait of Ramesh himself.

Ramesh has published several transcriptions of his talks on non-duality of the Advaita variety, and I'd heard of him and his living-room darshans from several different groups of friends. He's much thinner and much older than I anticipated, frail and birdlike, with the translucent, paper-thin skin that falls in on itself. He sits in a low-slung chair and is dressed all in white. I don't know if he's lost his top teeth or if, as he's aged — he is, after all, 91! — his upper palate has receded. As he talks, he produces small amounts of spittle, which he dabs away with a carefully folded white cloth kept on his lap for that purpose.

Ramesh's intellect is tack-sharp. As we enter, he grills a middle-aged Westerner seated in one of today's two "hot seats." These are the seats those with questions for Ramesh are asked to take.

A rotund Indian man slumps in an armchair that faces Ramesh and works a video camera on a tripod. The cameraman will occasionally pan from Ramesh to the questioner in the hot seat, and once or twice he pans around the room to capture the faces in the crowd.

Also facing Ramesh and seated just in front of us is a sound guy, an Indian fellow who works a professional-looking sound mixing board. He adjusts the levels and volume of the clip-on microphones attached to Ramesh and, on this day, to the two people sitting in the hot seats.

Arrayed on the coffee table in front of us are stacks of DVDs of previous talks, each labeled with titles like "Anger" or "Hate" or "Desire." After Ramesh's official talk ends, but before the 10 minutes of chanting begin that will close out the day, the camera guy will have mastered and burned copies of the day's talks. The sound guy murmurs to us that we can buy the DVD of our talk for 500 Rupees.

Ramesh has the probing mind of a brilliant debater, and quickly hones in on the actual question, which is often quite different than the one originally verbalized. When he addresses the questions — one couldn't really say he "answers" them — he espouses his ideas about reality, God, and consciousness.

According to Ramesh, if you look hard enough, long enough, you will come to realize that there is in fact no "doer." There is only Source. There is only Consciousness. Self-realization is the understanding that the "the doing" happens *through* us. In *Consciousness Writes*, Ramesh quotes Yang-Chu: 'Let the ear hear what it longs to hear.' When there is disassociation or dis-identification with whatever happens to the body-mind mechanism ... the prevailing tendencies of the body-mind are merely witnessed without any comparing or judging."

Days later, a friend asked me if I thought Ramesh had "It." I hemmed and hawed. I didn't know. I still don't know. Based on what Ramesh said, I would say he definitely had a taste. My personal understanding of Ramesh, and whether he has "It," is in the same vein as a Picasso anecdote, which I doubtless misremember: some time in the '30s the painter was accosted by a woman at a party who insisted that she neither understood nor cared much for Cubism. "But madam!" said Picasso. "It really doesn't matter!"

That day, on the way out, I notice a wall-length rack of books for sale written by Ramesh and his protégé Wayne Liquormann. I stop and browse. An Indian man, the proprietor, asks, "Yes! What books have you read?"

I point to the Ramesh titles I'd read before.

"Ah, then you need this one, this one, this one," he says, and puts one, two, three books in my hand. It's the hard sell.

I hand them back and say, "No, no thanks."

You can't blame people for wanting to get over. You can't knock the hustle. The cottage industry around Ramesh doesn't detract from his teaching. It sure makes for a surprising, surreal and unsavory experience.

HOW TO MAKE ASHTANGA VINYASA MORE DIFFICULT

Virtually all books on Yoga asana include copious instructions on how to scale down the postures. This is because 99 percent of us need it.

I did the very first forward bend of my life in my very first Yoga class at age 23. Any and all correct or misguided thoughts, memories, and imaginings crashed to an utter halt. There was only the grinding discomfort of the back of my legs, a nether region of whose existence I had never dreamt, let alone embodied with such excruciating immediacy.

But what if someone folds forward, slaps their forehead on their shins, and yawns? Let's talk about how to make practice more difficult.

To whom might this apply? In my experience, circus performers and former competitive gymnasts demonstrate the most complete range of active, dynamic and passive flexibility I have ever seen. They're rare in that their annamaya koshas, or "food bodies," are highly trained and conditioned due to years of daily, disciplined physical practices, and many if not all elements of Primary Series pale in comparison to the training they underwent as adolescents. Let's face it, Primary, Intermediate and most of the Advanced Series aren't a challenge to an 11-year-old with even 2 years of modern competitive gymnastic training.

During the practice for and performance of their routines, contortionists and gymnasts integrate the annamaya and pranamaya koshas, the food- and breath-bodies, and spend a fair amount of time absorbed in the latter limbs of pratyahara, dharana, dhyana, and samadhi.

For these people, the initial inherent challenge in Ashtanga is to simply practice the Primary Series until they've learned it by heart. The second challenge is to learn the prescribed breathing and transitions. A concrete and direct participation in inhale-up, exhale-down helps them shift to perhaps a more devotional and personal focus and away from a performance or competition mind-set, in which practice is only and merely a means to a much-delayed end.

Despite the simplicity and ease of the asana sequences, contortionists and gymnasts can develop a love for the rhythmic flow of the breath-body movement. They might also stick to the Ashtanga practice as they develop love and respect for their teacher. A heart-connection is a very powerful force that draws people to practice.

Either way, once their discipline and strength flows in this Yoga, and they learn the Primary Series, they will progress through the various series until they find a particularly interesting pebble in their shoe … which may only happen in the later (much later) series.

Richard Freeman has frequently observed that Pattabhi Jois was quite a trickster. During one trip to Mysore, when I practiced the Sunday led Intermediate classes, Guruji would have us hop up to a half-handstand after Vatayanasana … and then he would have us hover there. He would pad around the room, saying, "Why shaking?" and laughing.[5]

In this spirit, there are several ways to critically and subtly shift asanas and transitions of the first two series to make them

---

5 Rolf Naujokat later mentioned Jois was just "having fun."

compelling to a woman who can perform 10 L-sit press-handstands. Importantly, these small shifts still remain true to the traditional sequencing as well as ujjayi, asana and bandha, and drishti.

I have two fundamental principles I use when, for example, a recent Julliard grad discovers the Mysore practice. The first is rooted in physics: decrease leverage to increase resistance. This will greatly increase the difficulty of a vinyasa or asana, as well as hopefully increase the residual concentration, bandha engagement, sense-withdrawal, focus, and absorption.

The second principle I use is wedded to the first, and is what firmly ties any transition or posture to the tristana of Ashtanga Vinyasa. This principle is rooted in the pranamaya kosha: the inhale creates expansiveness and corresponds with prana, or upward-flowing sensation. The exhale corresponds with the apana, or the downward and rooting sensation. The technique of vinyasa, of synching breath and movement, yokes the different sides of the breath to the corresponding and complementary movement.

So I will look to decrease leverage while engaging the tristana. I can use surya namaskar A as an example, though the applications are endless. During the inhale (*trini* or three-count), one can press one's feet off the floor, legs as straight as possible. The legs swing up and open from the body. The straighter they are, the heavier the load.

I personally don't encourage press to full handstand for surya namaskar A and B. Full, deep ujjayi breathing is not possible in a properly vertically aligned handstand. (The banana handstand, yes, but that's a different handstand.) Balance becomes the prime focus, rather than ujjayi breathing, asana and bandha, and drishti, often with disastrous consequences for people practicing nearby. Also, the breath tends to stop entirely during a slow press up, which undercuts the vinyasa principle that girds this practice. Press handstands are discouraged in Mysore, India, and finally, regardless of the handstander's intent, the move can create a performance-based dynamic in a Mysore room.

So the transition to chaturanga dandasana should finish before the inhale stops, and this is generally what stops even the most Herculean person from pressing to handstand all over the place.

There are several transitions possible from the top of chaturanga dandasana to urdvha mukkha svasana, and from there to adho mukkha svasana. Chaturanga dandasana becomes more interesting as the triceps approach parallel and the wrists approach the waist. Just a small movement of the hands in this direction greatly lessens leverage.

The triceps, chest and front delts are severely taxed, and there's a full contraction of the lats, mid- and low-back as well as the traps. The triceps and the forearms fire like crazy to stabilize the elbow joint. The bandhas are absolutely enlivened as the upper and lower abs, obliques, serratus, the muscles of the pelvic floor, and the hip flexors all struggle to keep the hips level with the shoulders.

This migration of the wrists toward the waist should be gradual, as not only is muscular strength built but the connective tissue is conditioned.

The movement from upward-facing dog to downward-facing dog is made more engaging by reversing the entrance. That is, by rolling back down to the bottom of chaturanga dandasana as though rolling under a bar, and then, elbows close in, by pressing up into downward-facing dog. Chuck Miller demonstrates this method, also known as a dive-bomber push-up, in the 1993 Yoga Works videos.

It is vital to inhale-up, exhale-back. If the breath becomes strained or stops, the transition is too much for the person and should be adjusted so the breath flows. As I've heard Pattabhi Jois quoted (in turn quoting Patanjali's *Yoga Sutras* I.31): "Breath shaking, body shaking ... mind shaking!"

The move from downward-facing dog back to standing mirrors the entrance: one begins the inhale and then hops, with straight legs, to lower the feet between the hands. The inhale carries through and, fingertips on the floor, raises the head.

Uth pluthi, like surya namaskar another pose practiced daily, can become much more interesting when one adopts an L-shape rather than a curled-C. I came to appreciate this when, during led class, Sharath Rangaswamy would say, "Don't touch your legs to your arms!" If I press my center of gravity forward from my base of support — my hands — a decrease in leverage of mere centimeters increases the resistance exponentially.

The first two series also feature jump-backs from seated asanas. To decrease leverage, practice the inhale-up-lolasana with straight legs in an L-shape prior to the exhale back to chaturanga.

My progression for jump-backs and jump-thrus begins with the easiest — the straight-leg hinge at the hips. From there, move from bent legs/crossed shins to bent legs/side-by-side shins.

Additionally, one is always stronger in a bent-arm position. Unfortunately there's very little carryover from bent-arm to straight-arm strength. So if someone can consistently jump back and jump thru for the entire Primary Series with bent arms, and can also jump back after 25 breaths in uth pluthi, it's time to develop straight-arm strength.

I'd recommend this practitioner jump back and jump thru and maintain completely straight arms the entire time. Straight-arm strength is also developed during the transitions into and out of bhujapidasana, supta kurmasana, and dwi pada sirsasana. It's also built moving into, out of, and during the states of bakasana A and B and tittibasana. At no point are the arms to bend — meaning, don't start with bent arms and then straighten them while in the pose.

In this way, the transitions of even the Primary Series becomes incredibly compelling to contortionists and gymnasts alike, and yet remain grounded in ujjayi breathing, the asanas, which incorporate the bandhas, and the drishti. Movement is yoked to breath and the practice becomes a vital, sensual dance.

After uth pluthi, everyone — gymnast, contortionist, and stiff white guy alike — sit, breathe, and take rest, and invite the profound, splendid stillness that is the inevitable and incredible byproduct of the Ashtanga Vinyasa practice.

ASHTANGA YOGA JOURNAL EDIT MEETING NOTES

Notes from a recent *Ashtanga Yoga Journal* editorial meeting:

Proposed Article Topics:
Pattabhi Jois: Always Right or Simply Never Wrong?
Coffee Before Intermediate: Good or Bad?
Investigative Report: Does Ashtanga Make Women Hard and Men Soft?
Men's Fashion — Banana Hammocks Versus Board Shorts

Reader Poll Ideas:
Shala Voted Best Place to Meet Cute Guys; Knee Pain: Symptomatic or Asymptomatic?; Romantic Advice: Fending Off Creepy Male Ashtangis; Breaking Up: Who Gets the Shala?
"Mars and Venus in the Shala" (note: GENIUS!)
Best Pre-tan Tips Before Hitting Southern Star
Beauty in the Shala: Makeup That Won't Run When You Sweat
NY Scene Report: Best People Watching; Best Post-practice Dosa; Celebrity Spotting
Essay: Ashtanga — Not Just for Hippies Anymore

Proposed Cover Shots for June/July

(Note to photog: prefer sharp photo to blurry, poorly framed digi/instant)

Pattabhi Jois smiling
Pattabhi Jois grinning
Pattabhi Jois laughing
Pattabhi Jois waving
Pattabhi Jois counting a led class

Additional notes:

—Not enough space for entirety of Richard Freeman's asana advice column — publish separately as 300-page book?

—Tell art director NOT to Photoshop hair onto Swenson's head!

—Potential ad buys? Have reps call: Ibuprofen, Motrin, Ben Gay, Tiger Balm, Starbuck's, all imported chocolate manufacturers.

YANAL CONTROL

I'm not really that smart. I have a mind for minutiae, a steel-trap for trivia, but I'm not quick on the uptake when it comes to translating abstract Yoga concepts into everyday experience.

Which means I greatly admire the poetry of directions like "Lift your kidneys," "Open your heart," or "Practice non-attachment." Like, I get it. But only intellectually. Looking back at my experience in various led-class Yoga asana settings, directives like those immediately established in me a glaring gap between what I was experiencing and what I thought I should be feeling. Like I said, maybe it's my own faulty wiring, but I don't know how to "open my heart."

The instances when I've had great heart openings have never been intentional, and they've always arisen independent of my own desires or efforts.

What was worse, for me aphorisms like the ones above helped build a model of experience separate from my own, which turned the practice of Yoga into my efforts to get to, achieve, or attain that model.

Over time, what grounded me were the mundane and decidedly simple physical (and thereby mental and spiritual) Yoga techniques that I could actually *do*: Inhale, exhale. Activate mula bandha, or "Take yanal control," as Pattabhi Jois used to say.[6]

To have a goal or intention is okay. This is what the bandhas do for my ujjayi breath: they anchor and give shape and direction to the in- and out-breath. It's okay to want to perform an asana, or even get better at it. To paraphrase Zen teacher Shunryu Suzuki: make the effort, then lose yourself in the effort. For me, it's that perpetual return to the breath, bandhas, and gazing points that allow the non-attachment and heart-opening to arise. Or not.

Yoga practice becomes an engagement with what I can do, and this relationship with what I can do *right now* is an engagement and relationship with the boring splendor of everyday, ordinary reality.

---

[6] Regarding the book *Mula Bandha: The Master Key*, my thoughts on the subject currently are this: if you can stop the flow of urine and feces, you are intimately familiar with mula bandha. Otherwise, what use?

SARTORIAL SPLENDOR

As the editor and writer of the world's leading Ashtanga Yoga blog, I am frequently asked by the editors of various fashion magazines — *Elle*, *Bazaar*, *Dazed and Confused*, *Vogue* (both US *and* British versions), *W*, and *Cat Fancy* — how my current Yoga look has evolved. Tom Ford, for example, dubbed my fall/winter 2006 look "The Yogi Roué."

So loyal readers, here's the same sartorial story my publicist faxes annually to those august publications. It's the story of my various industry-changing looks.

The outfit at my first Yoga class ever consisted of a t-shirt and sweatpants, both cotton. During this first class, so much sweat geysered from every pore on my body that I soaked completely through both pants and shirt. What happens when you exceed your garments' sweat-carrying capacity? Why, your sweat funnels into deep and embarrassing pools on the Yoga studio floor. One would assume that sweatpants are in fact "pants" to be "sweated" in. Certainly, however, they were never designed to be sweated *through*.

Yoga asana did more than establish me as a profligate all-body sweater. My first class, at some studio on Sunset in Los Angeles' Los Feliz neighborhood, was also noteworthy because, while the we rested in savasana, the teacher read aloud a section from an animal rights book that described, in graphic detail, how pigs were killed at a slaughterhouse. Restful stuff!

In subsequent Yoga classes I unveiled my "casual skateboarder" look: board shorts and wife-beater. I had one pair of board shorts (dark blue, Stüssy) that had a 36-inch waist. My waist size was several inches less than that. Consequently my crack twinkled at any unfortunate classmates behind me. Additionally, I only washed these shorts once a week.[7]

Going shirtless in public was not something I ever anticipated, but I continued to be a pornographic sweat-hog, so eventually I had to shed the wife-beater. I would sweat through every square inch of it. It was like wearing a wet newspaper.

This was in San Francisco, so believe it or not, my sandwich-bread-flat ass, its attendant crack, and my shorts' musky scent[8] went largely unnoticed at our local studio, which was situated in the heart of the Mission district. Let's just say that Ahimsa Yoga attracted some rather interesting personalities.

For example, I once or twice practiced next to a fellow my age who wore baggy full-length raver-style blue jeans. He emitted the distinctive and pungent ether tang of crystal methamphetamine. His sweat was also a crusty, jaundice-yellow color.

Eventually I lost my Stussy boardshorts, so I upgraded to dark blue gym shorts I got for $6 a pair at a sports outlet store. They were cotton. You think I would have learned not to mess with cotton at this point, but no. I would also sweat entirely through these shorts.

It should be obvious that, at this point, sweat management was paramount to my Yoga practice. Ways in which to collect, funnel, transport and then disperse the prodigious and surprising amount of water produced was a topic of great concern to me. It required serious infrastructure, as my Yoga wardrobe needed to

---

[7] I lie. It was significantly less than that.

[8] Which, I maintain, has a fantastic bouquet that is at worst intensely pleasurable and at best a powerful aphrodisiac.

account for channeling, wicking, and sluicing of unceasing torrents.

So the cotton gym shorts were a failure. Their other drawback was that they required boxer-briefs underneath, or else the class was treated to either full-frontal or sidepipe shots.

I still wasn't ready to jump into spandex-type shorts, though, so I invested the ungodly sum of $40 in a pair of Nike runners' shorts. They were synthetic, and unlike the cotton gym shorts, didn't feel like wet papier mache an hour into class. They also featured an inner lining that gathered up and lovingly cocooned my cash and prizes from the ever-prying eyes of Yoga babes.

Unfortunately, disaster struck. I lost this pair. The cotton gym shorts also proved disadvantageous as, over time, the constant shimmying, prancing, and cavorting that took place during my Yoga asana practice resulted in the drastic stretching of all three pairs. I could handle a bit of stretch around the waist ... but the *leg holes* were stretching, too, which led to warranted anxiety that one day, during class, Big Jim and the Twins would burst forth, unbidden, like a sand-worm in *Dune*.

At this point I abandoned all sense of shame. I went to Swooshtown and plunked down $70 for two pairs of tight, form-fitting matte-black running shorts made of material used on the space shuttle. When I say these shorts were tight, I mean *tight* — grape-smugglers, banana hammocks, meat-pockets, jewel-bags, coin-purses. It had been a long journey to spandex, or at least a high-tech spandex derivative, but I had arrived.

When I say "spandex," I think of the Big Guns in those '93 Yoga Works videos. I love those videos, and not just because El Gran Jefe Tim Miller shines as a bronzed, muscled alien crash-landed among sun-starved twig-men and hairy-pitted women, the latter unsexed in shapeless unitards. No, I love those videos because all the dudes' spandex shorts were color-coordinated.

Watching those old videos, as well as others, you get a sense that, despite the many companies that have sprouted up to sell us cooler and more (or less) athletic Yoga wear, what really matters at the end of the day are functional clothes.[9]

Maybe I'm in the middle of a clothing parabola. At this stage, I alternate between spandex and running shorts. But maybe, as I get older and fatter, I'll begin to bundle up again, reversing the evolution. I'll move from tight shorts into cotton gym shorts, and then board-shorts, and finally, in my old age, I'll once again soak through cotton sweat-pants and a white t-shirt screen-printed with that classic koan "Who Farted?"

---

[9] Of course, how functional is *too* functional? There was a lovely couple in Mysore who both wore such short-shorts that the lower quarter-moons of their ass-cheeks jiggled, rippled and bobbled for those of us behind them. Guruji used to say, "Keep your mind on God!" I tried to think of God but kept getting ass-cheek. I tried to think of the ass-cheeks as God. It didn't work. I switched spots.

RHIZOMATIC ASHTANGA

What if the eight limbs weren't a tree?
What if they were a root?

A rhizome is a "root-like, subterranean stem, commonly horizontal in position, that usually produces roots below and sends up shoots progressively from the upper surface." Ginger is a rhizome. So at first, a conception of Ashtanga Vinyasa Yoga as rhizomatic seems counterintuitive, because the common metaphor of the "eight limbs" is the image of a tree, vertical and growing skyward, aboveground.

A rhizome, on the other hand, is the inversion of this: it's horizontal and underground.

According to Gilles Deleuze and Félix Guattari, who conceived of the rhizome concept, an "arborescent" tree-and-root metaphor uses dualist categories and forces us to make binary choices. Connections are vertical and linear. In *A Thousand Plateaus*, the two philosophers also suggest that a root-tree system forces us to use an arrow of time model. It charts cause-and-effect (karma!) along chronological lines. This model of thinking causes us to look back for the source of "things" and forward to the end of those "things."

An arborescent map of spiritual practice is implicit in the yogic systems that emphasize awakening the kundalini in the base of the spine, which is then raised chronologically, vertically and linearly upward through the chakras, to finally reach the pinnacle, the sahasrara chakra, at the top.

The root-tree way of thinking has its shortcomings. It imposes an artificial linearity on an organic process and system. It also creates a narrator, someone separate from the passage of time and to whom events occur.

On the other hand, rather than turning history, culture and spiritual practices into a story with an observer-narrator, the rhizome presents "a map or array of attractions and influences with no specific origin or genesis." For Delueze and Guattari, a "rhizome has no beginning or end; it is always in the middle, between things, interbeing, intermezzo." It "resists chronology and organization, and instead favors a nomadic system of growth and propagation."

How can we take a rhizomatic look at Ashtanga? In Ashtanga Vinyasa and indeed Ashtanga Yoga, one can start with any limb. The system has multiple and non-hierarchical entrances and exits, as one has often already always been practicing or embodying specific limbs.

We can turn the image of a vertical tree on its side and bury it in the earth, and the eight limbs become eight roots that twist and turn on each other, growing, thickening, connected to and containing each other. The yamas and niyamas feed and inform each other, in turn to feed and inform asana and pranayama. To paraphrase Deleuze and Guattari, a rhizomatic conception of Ashtanga Vinyasa turns us toward a "ceaseless establishment of connections."

In other words, toward a ceaseless establishment of Yoga.

LILLIAN

I met Lillian in Encinitas. At one point, our breakfast conversation drifted to past indiscretions, excesses and indulgences, and how we'd found Yoga. She'd had her road-to-Damascus moment in the bathroom of a downtown San Diego dive bar at 4 a.m. She had stared at herself in the mirror, coked to the gills and holding a bloody chunk of septum in her right hand.

Not everyone is like Saul of Tarsus. One day, while traveling to Damascus, Saul saw a blinding light and heard quite clearly the voice of God. He was pitched to the ground from his horse and arose to become Paul, one of the more ardent early Christians. Not everyone is pitched from his or her horse by the voice of God. Sometimes the call is a faint, ghostly echo, hard to hear over the bass thud of the club speakers or the dull roar of party conversation.

The night Lillian heard her own call, she'd partied pretty hard on Wednesday and Thursday nights, caught very little sleep in between, then dove back in on Friday night. That weekend the party train hit all stops, from bar to club, club to after-hours, after-hours back to bar. Friday night strobed into early Sunday morning and the last stop was Gentleman Jack's, a downtown San Diego dive, small, cramped, dark, seedy.

Saturday night at 2 a.m. the bartender swept out the crowd. He locked the front door, pulled the blinds, killed the lights, turned up the jukebox, and dumped large, chunky off-white rocks of cocaine on the bar. One of Lillian's friends pulled out a hand coffee-grinder and started churning the rocks into powder. Everyone took turns hoovering finger-thick rails straight off the bar.

Four a.m. Sunday morning and Lil was in the bathroom, wiping the drip from her nose. Her heart was revved so high it felt like a fist thumping her breastbone from inside. And her nose! It itched, bad. She had a booger or a hair that just would not quit. Lillian closed off one nostril and with a firm snort blew a thick, blood-red chunk of scab into her hand. It was a piece of her septum.

"Beyond a certain point there is no return," said Kafka. "This point has to be reached." A piece of her nose in hand, Lil had a flash-panic anxiety attack. At that point, her point of no return, three thoughts surfaced, clear and crystal and pure as a polished diamond: "I need to stop partying," followed by "I need to get healthy or I'm going to die," and finally, "I need to start doing Yoga."

Lillian doesn't know where the last thought came from. Maybe she'd read about Yoga somewhere? Regardless, the seed had been planted. She sifted those three realizations, swirled and rinsed them, until she found Ashtanga Vinyasa Yoga.

Today Lillian is strong, healthy and vibrant. Radiant, even.

ASHTANGA AT ALTITUDE

"If some people are telling you they had their climax on Mount Everest, they lied," says Reinhold Messner[10]. "It is an awful place."

Why risk everything to go there?

"Without the possibility of death," Messner replied, "adventure is not possible."

Messner is hailed as the world's greatest mountaineer. He ascended, with longtime partner Peter Habeler, the 26,470-foot summit of Gasherbrum I, called Hidden Peak, in 1975. It's one of the giants of the Himalayas. Most remarkable of all, though, was that Messner and Habeler ascended without porters, camps, fixed ropes, or oxygen.

They then scaled Everest without oxygen in May 1978, a feat that National Geographic says "took climbing to the absolute limit." Three months later, Messner climbed Nanga Parbat, the ninth highest mountain on Earth, solo. Two years later, he again climbed Mount Everest without oxygen, equipped with a single small rucksack — and alone.

---

[10] *National Geographic,* **November 2006**

Messner was the first climber to ascend all 14 "eight-thousanders," or peaks over 8,000 meters tall.

The Yoga of Messner's climbing, and make no mistake, it is Yoga, involves intense practice and dedication. "If I am well-prepared," says Messner, "and if I'm living a long time in my visions, in my fantasy, with my challenge, before doing it, I'm living with it, I'm dreaming about it, planning, preparing, training."

The residue of his practice is a fierce, consuming, and single-pointed state of concentration. "So when I start to climb," he continues, "especially when I'm on a big wall, whatever the difficulties — I'm so concentrated that there is nothing else existing; there's only a few meters of wall where I am hanging and climbing; and in this concentration, everything seems quite logical. There is no danger anymore. The danger is gone ... But the concentration is absolute."

As Messner says, without the possibility of death, adventure is not possible. It must be understood, however, that for Messner, the idea of "life" and "adventure" are inextricably intertwined, for it is true, too, that without the possibility of death, life is not possible. In this case, "life" is opposite to the idea of subsistence, which is the ceaseless reaction to external stimuli — avoiding discomfort, seeking its opposite — eternally buffeted by the mind's internal chatter and its cherished anxieties and neuroses.

For Messner, that internal chatter is stilled in the face of absolute danger, a danger for which he has rigorously practiced.

"There are moments in difficult situations, far away, that there is no more doubt," he says. "There, the questions are gone. And I think these are the important moments. If the question is gone, I have not to answer. Myself living — I am the answer."

Messner has paid heavy dues to the mountains: frostbite claimed five toes and three fingers, and during his first Himalayan expedition in 1970, Nanga Parbat claimed the life of his younger brother Gunther.

Is it possible to become Messner's "myself living," to become one's own "answer," without stumbling to the summit of

Everest, half-mad with oxygen deprivation, at the edge of starvation and dehydration?

MYSORE 2005

Straight from the Tap

The milk boy delivers fresh milk, still warm from the udder, every day at 4:30 p.m. for the sum of 7 rupees. We've bought a one-liter milk pail expressly for the purpose. The milk boy pours out a half-liter into our pail, and then, with a well-practiced, graceful Mobius swirl of the wrist, dips his cup back into the bucket to top it off.

The milk boy does, however, walk directly into our living room without knocking. He doesn't stand in the hallway, doorway, or even inside the general front-door area. The door will suddenly swing wide and he'll troop into the living room.[11]

Andrew boils the milk for 2 to 3 minutes; it usually ends up foamed for cappuccino, although I've been known to pour a bowl for cereal.

---

[11] We canceled our milk delivery service when one day the milk boy entered our house and tried to touch Tara. I was showering at the time and came out when I heard Tara calling for help. Nude, I escorted the milk boy out of our house and down the steps.

Mysore's Subtle Tyranny

Be free from the idea that you must only read books about Yoga! Liberate yourself from the creeping anxiety that your free time must consist of chanting, Sanskrit and Sutra classes! Read John Grisham, Michael Crichton, Stephen King, Tom Clancy, Frederick Forsythe, Robert Ludlum! Rent and watch films you would never dream of watching! *American Pie 3*! *40-Year-Old Virgin*! *Orgazmo*!

Casual Piracy

Video Tech is on Kalidasa Road, across from the petrol station. I have to duck my head to enter its open garage-door storefront. Hundreds of VCDs line the four walls, while the more expensive DVDs are tucked in a small recessed alcove behind the front counter.

I'm sure I pay Westerner prices, or 30Rs per DVD, so the kid working the desk lets me behind the counter to squat on a stool to sort through the good shit. He even turns on an overhead bulb for me. There's *Wedding Crashers*, *Fantastic Four*, *War of the Worlds*, *Red Eye*, and incongruously, Renoir's *The Grand Illusion*.

There's a 1-in-10 chance my laptop simply won't read the DVD. Many copies are filmed directly off the screen. We've been fortunate, though, as none of the copies we've rented have included filmgoers' heads, though *Wedding Crashers* had an audience laugh-track.

I also sort through a basket of music CDs on the counter. You can rent them for 15Rs each per day. One CD contained 15 Pink Floyd albums, another had 11 Metallica albums, and the last contained 13 of the latest pop albums (Backstreet Boys, Jennifer Lopez, Black Eyed Peas, The Scorpions, Richard Marx.)

Also courtesy of Video Tech, last week we watched 21 episodes from the third season of *Seinfeld*, and on Sunday the entire first season of *Sex and the City*. Decadent? Maybe. Downright sybaritic? One could make the case.

Lakshmipuram Organic Market

From our flat in Gokulam we scooter through the Mysore University grounds to the Lakshmipuram neighborhood. Rowan is 1; Tara wears her in a frontal sling and sits behind me on our scooter. In a fluorescent Styrofoam helmet that engulfs her baby head, Rowan looks like a human pushpin. The helmet slips down over her eyes, so she uses her delicate baby hands to hold it up in order to survey the scenery. Andrew pilots the other scooter, Allison on back, her long blonde hair trailing in the wind. We are an eye-catching bunch.

The street intensity ratchets upwards during the drive. Lakshmipuram is more compact, tighter, louder, and more concentrated than Gokulam.

Andrew has found the location of the organic market he frequented on his first trip to Mysore, back in 2001. The market is now in a rundown, mould-covered house, in which the "market" takes up one walk-in closet-sized room. Weevils sit in sacks of dal; spiders leap from bunches of bananas. Andrew buys organic mung dal, liquid jaggery, organic coffee, and some honey. Allison stocks up on greens.

Tara and I take Rowan out front. Her blonde hair and translucent skin are an instant hit with the Indian men sitting around the entrance. One man is an endless font of folk medicine: One drop of honey on the baby's tongue per morning, he says, will make her learn to talk better, faster. For teething pain, rub sugar on her gums.

We show baby Rowan to the cow that grazes across the street. "Woof, woof," says Rowan, which is what she says when she sees any animal. A piece of rope ties the cow's neck to its front foreleg so that it can't raise its head more than 2 feet from the ground.

The folk-medicine man tells us the cow is so dumb that it will walk into and through cars, people, and glass windows. Therefore its gaze is roped down. I'd never seen a live farm animal until India, so I'm very much out of my depth.

Andrew and Allison finish shopping, and we scooter back to Gokulam. Later, Andrew uses his new coffee in my stovetop espresso maker. When the moka pot begins hissing, Andrew lifts the lid. "Look," he says, "it's boiling out like cream!" And he's right. The organic coffee foams through the slit like cream.

Getting Internet

Andrew bought two Apple iSight cameras prior to coming to India, one for my Mac, one for his wife's Mac. This way he would be able to see and talk to her and his 2-year-old son.

We fished two Internet service provider contact names from the Internet place around the corner and called them. "No connection is possible in your neighborhood," the first place told us.

We met with a representative from the second place. They wanted a 10,000 Rupee deposit. They had once hooked up broadband for a Western Yoga student, and the student had made 30,000 Rupees-worth of long-distance calls before vanishing back to the West.

Our landlady's son Dutt intervened. They put the connection in their name, and therefore, no deposit and no installation fee.

We return from Yoga practice one day to find an amorphous swarm of workers, numbering not less than eight and not more than 11, chopping up the street the length of the entire block in order to lay the cable for our Internet connection. The squad worked for four or five hours, and then vanished as they'd appeared.

Now the cable is laid, though the Internet does not function, as it will be some weeks before we circumnavigate both the language barrier and Byzantine Indian business practices to get it turned on.

In front of the house, and in front of the line of workers, I loan Andrew 100 Rupees, separating the bill from others like it in my wallet. I realize too late I have just flashed a week's wages or more to the dark, sun-creased men who pickaxe the dirt.

Slapstick Karma

I pursue a mosquito in our living room, and I slip on a throw rug and sprain my wrist.

The Yoga

Each morning, Tara and I leave Rowan with Nirmala, our landlady, who has agreed to watch Rowan six days a week, two hours a day, for 1,000 Rs. a month. Guruji has asked us to arrive at 5:30, and during the last week-and-a-half we've entered the studio to an ever-increasing number of floor vacancies as attendance has dwindled.

The density in my back and shoulders, which accreted during six weeks of crisscrossing the U.S. via planes, trains and automobiles, has started to melt. My body unkinked from the flight sometime last week. I had been having strong and light practices; then, one day, I felt grounded, strong and light.

Guruji is 90 and fiery. He pads about the room, squat and powerful, shouting, his eyes twinkling. Last week he suffered from a deep, wet cough, but it seems to have cleared.

Tara, Andrew and I (and Rowan) registered together, and Guruji demanded to know when our teacher Tim Miller would be arriving. I lamely replied, "December?" because it seemed a fair guess.

Guruji shuffled our stacks of money into an electronic money counter, which immediately conjured images of the last few places I'd seen the device, namely at the homes of my drug-dealer acquaintances and in the movie *Scarface*. The machine whirred and beeped when it had processed our stack of Rupee notes.

So: show up early, breathe, move. There are moments of an emptiness so full, a silence so loud I only notice them when they've passed.

I did not bow my head to Guruji's feet on my last trip. Not once. This time it is different. There is a swelling, expansive gratitude that inflates deep in my chest and pushes tears into my eyes. I do the logical and illogical thing and touch his feet. For how fortunate I am to inhabit this body and to have found this practice! Guruji laughs and says, "Tankew, tankew," as though I do him a favor.

GOA 2008

Why We Moved Out of Our Flat
"There's a mouse in the pool, Daddy," the kid tells me.
"A mouse?"
"Yes, Daddy, a mouse! A! Mouse!" She says the last bit slowly, plaintively, making sure I understand. Tara and I had done the Kid Handoff at the Yoga studio, and Rowan and I had just pulled into the driveway of our flat.

Sure enough, she's right. There is a mouse in the pool. The "pool," in this case, is a small decorative fountain at the head of the driveway, and serves as the centerpoint for the two flats and the large garden that make up our little compound. A short palm hangs leafy arms over a pedestal with a statue of Mary on it, and Mary in turn looks down on the water of the fountain, which is about 5 feet around and a foot deep, with a knee-high lip. In the otherwise all-white bottom sits an incongruous maple leaf design made from blue tile pieces. The 18-inch Mary statue has been placed in a large glass ampule, as though a giant will amble past and toss back the mother of Christ like an ibuprofen.

Queenie Fernandes, the owner of the property, has three turtles that she lets flap around in the pond. The lip is high enough that there's no risk they might climb out. The turtles have thick red swatches around their eyes, which you can see when they extend their heads from their shells. They do this when Rowan and I lean over and try to pet them. They're fearless turtles, apparently, and it's almost like they want to be petted. Queenie feeds them puffed rice, and once a week lets them eat some meat.

The turtles are only allowed in the fountain when Queenie is at home, though. "People will come to steal them," she tells me. "I can't leave them in there without someone around."

On the day Rowan spies a "mouse," however, the turtles are not in the pool. And Rowan hasn't actually seen a mouse, of course. It's a dead rat. Its bloated foot-and-a-half-long body circles aimlessly in the water.

The rodent must've fallen into the pool during the night and, unable to claw its way over the lip, drowned. I left for practice when it was still dark, so I hadn't seen it that morning.

Goa was for a long time a Portuguese colony, and the Portuguese influence is writ large across this part of India, from the Spanish surnames and churches to the Christianity and the architecture. Many houses are built with front-gabled roofs covered with red tiles. The roofs slant upwards at a 45-degree angle on either side to meet in the center. This is different than, say, Mysore, where most houses have flat roofs. Inside many Goa houses the ceilings are unfinished, so you can see the underside of the tiles.

In our flat there was perhaps a foot of overlap where the roof hung over the walls, which meant there was open space through which the heat as well as moths, mosquitoes and flies could pass.

In our bedroom, part of the ceiling tiling had been replaced with sheets of corrugated tin. We would wake several times in the night to the *tik-tik-tik* of paws scraping across the roof, paws doubtless belonging to 2-foot-long rats. At least twice a night there would be a loud *bang!* as something big and heavy jumped on the tin. Dust, dirt and leaves would flutter down on our beds. Tara and I would lie there and stare upward, listening for whatever hit the roof to make its way into the house. I began sleeping with a broomstick next to the bed.

One morning, after I had gone to Yoga, Tara was awoken by a panicked rattling in the kitchen. She woke up Rowan, and the two of them stood outside the darkened kitchen as something rocketed about, trying to find a way out.

"Mommy was freaking out," said Rowan. Tara hurled a few empty water jugs into the kitchen, and whatever was there managed to find its way back out. That was it. We moved out. We're spending our last week at Resort Melo Rosa, a modest, rat-free hotel.

I tend to be fairly ambivalent about pests. As long as I'm asleep when they're around, I'm good. But Tara does not like rats (or snakes), and by "does not like," I mean "is terrified of." But you gotta draw the line somewhere, and really, finding rat droppings in our bedroom was the final straw.

The day that Rowan and I found the dead rat in the fountain, we returned from breakfast to find that Queenie had thrown the turtles into the fountain. The turtles gnaw on the dead rat, worrying out bloody chunks with their beaked mouths.

The turtles got their meat a little early that week. Rowan and I no longer reach out to pet them.

Know Your Goans

Bear with me for several dangerous over-generalizations about subcultures in Goa, India. There are roughly three large types that rocket past on motorbikes, clog restaurants and beaches, and stumble home on the roadside, wildly inebriated.

First, there's a dwindling population of hippies who washed ashore Back in the Day and never left. They tend to be a bit older, aged somewhere in their Fifties and Sixties, and their skin has tanned and cured into a terrific beef-jerky consistency. They might wear orange fisherman pants and a yellow kurta covered in "Om" symbols. Frequently you'll spot them wearing all white.[12]

---

[12] It is so goddamn hot, though, that I find myself eyeing loose, billowy, white India-style shirts and fisherman pants every time we go out. They look so comfortable, though both Tara and I have a standing policy not to buy clothes we can't and won't wear anywhere else in the world.

Next there are the crusties. These are extras from Mad Max's Thunderdome, the Babylon rave scene in *Matrix Reloaded,* or any movie made in the '90s about The Future. Remember, in the Future of the '90s we will all have dreadlocks, wear black vinyl clothing, and listen to techno. Crusties are of indeterminate nationality. They seem to favor Royal Enfields, those big bikes with the shiny silver carburetor boxes that make a distinctive pop-pop-pop engine sound.

Crusties' distinguishing characteristics include fierce black dreads that reach down to the ass, (which I imagine an incredible comfort in 30-degree-Celsius weather), as well as tribal tattoos, piercings, and other body-mods such as scarification and branding. Crusties tend to wear torn, tattered and multi-layered clothes assembled from the surplus uniforms of the world's various armies. The more utility pockets and/or leather, the better.

Finally, there are the tourists. You can spot them fairly easily 'cause they look fucking *lost*, out-of-place and sunburned wherever they are. Different beaches have been established as the home-base for different tourist nationalities. There's a British beach, as well as Russian and Israeli beaches. The corpulent Brits, their accents swallowing their syllables, trundle about with fists full of cheap cans of lager. Their skin is skunk-striped fishbelly white *and* radioactive red.

The Russian beaches seem the same as the British beaches, only more so: the men are fatter and paler, and yet they wear skimpier Speedo swimsuits. Many of the women on their arms are thin, blonde and beautiful. I'm later informed that this is not as incongruous as it first seems, as many of the women are prostitutes who live in Goa in Russian Mafia-run towns.

Many of the Israelis we meet are younger, early 20s, and are interesting and engaging, though many have just finished mandatory military service and are looking to get wasted with a zeal and determination bordering on the religious.

There's also a nascent subculture of "Yoga tourist" into which our family fits, and although this subculture is growing, it's small enough that it hasn't developed identifiable characteristics.

There are young couples, single moms, and young families. The average age range seems Twenties to Thirties, though I chalk that up to the fact that we're practicing Ashtanga Vinyasa. We didn't explore the different presentations of Yoga available in Goa, such as the devotional or sitting-based, chiefly because many of the publicized classes are held at more expensive resort or retreat centers.

Chapora Juice Bar

Head due west from the Barat Petroleum Station (as the sign says, "Pure For Sure!") in Anjuna toward Vagator Beach. Just prior to hitting the water, take a right and dive down a steep, winding canyon road to Chapora, where three roads meet under the boughs of a giant tree to form the heart of this tiny town. The tree is the ground-zero from which a cluster of small tourist shops has pulsed outward. The three streets are crammed with stalls that sell unique Goa clothing, an improbable collection of military surplus, day-glo fluorescence, and tie-dyed organic Nepalese hemp. There are also travel agencies, tour organizers, long-distance phone booths, and guest rooms.

Immediately under the large tree's trunk, on a small stage that rings all sides, sits a small Shiva shrine. The tree's trunk has been painted, and is decorated with malas and garlands.

The Chapora Juice Bar is within arm's reach of the stage. It's small and typically Indian, cramped, busy, dirty, utilitarian, and for those reasons it's anomalous among Goa's more polished and refined eateries. It's a small, square concrete building with a sliding front window through which one can order a variety of fresh juices and milkshakes. The menu has been hand-painted on the wall above the order window. Picnic tables sit in front and to the side of the building. Armies of flies hover, drawn by the fruit and the sugar.

Friends suggested the Juice Bar as an interesting hangout, so we visited on several occasions. It's quite popular, I think in part because it's a Goa rarity that offers genuine Indian prices. Juices range from 10 to 30 Rupees, which is a far cry from the 70 to 100 Rupee offerings at the nearby Bean Me Up.

Sit there long enough and you can watch tides of people wash in and out as the sun arcs overhead. During our visits we watched sadhus arrive, one by one, to take seats on the stage or at the picnic tables. Their gaunt bodies were wrapped in traditional orange sheets, their faces painted, and their dreads hung down to their waists. Curiously, all were white Westerners.

Many other Juice Bar frequenters were older, sun-leathered hippie ex-pats. One of whom, a Spanish gentleman, told Tara he arrived in Goa 25 years ago and simply threw away his passport. Many, faces ill-used and sun-cured, smiles revealing large gaps of missing teeth, look like they'd lived hard lives under a relentless tropical sun.

The actual juice at the Juice Bar is incidental to the place's appeal, which seemed to be marijuana, and it was around the weed that all seating arrangements at the picnic tables were based. Younger visitors commingled with the older residents, and at table after table it was quickly determined who had the mota, who had the chillum, and who could pack the best bowl.

The other, darker element at the Juice Bar, though, were those visitors, both younger and older, looking for more serious hook-ups. The most obvious had pale, spotty skin, dark circles under their eyes, and ceaseless sniffles. A girl who couldn't have been out of her early twenties sat in a corner, knees pulled in to her chest, and alternated between chewing a thumbnail and scratching at her arms, neck and legs.

Goa has a very dark side, one that seems out of place in the sun and sand, and yet is inevitable given both the 24-hour party scene here and India's overall exoticism. The exchange rate means many Westerners suddenly have vast wealth at their disposal, and to take a Westerner and unseat them from the deep structures of family, job, friends, language, and culture, and deposit them somewhere far, far away from the persona they inhabited, is to knock away any center of personal gravity and any psychic and psychological mooring.

Sprinkle on top of this the concept of "vacation" and "holiday," or "gap year" and "spiritual journey," and you have two recipes: the first for an anything-goes mentality in which every problem can be solved by throwing Rupees at it, or ultimately and decisively solved by boarding a plane home in two weeks. The second is a recipe for the Holy Mother India mentality, replete with its exoticism and fetishization.

Simply put, you can come to India and lose your goddamned mind.

It doesn't matter if you're in the shrill idleness of the tree-lined streets of Gokulam, in Mysore, with its mansions and incessant Yoga drone, or whether you're among the party-burnout transience on the sun-drenched beaches of Goa.

While in Mysore, I heard Sharath say, joking, "Do the Yoga. Now go home!" This is a sentiment echoed by my wife, whose sweet pragmatism keeps me from both internal and external withdrawal and renunciation.

Our last week in Goa, I took to guzzling ice-cold cans of Pepsi as though the brown sugar-syrup were some lifeline to familiarity. One afternoon we lay in bed, waiting out the heat. Tara rolled a cold can across my forehead, stroked my cheek gently and said, "Okay honey, it's time to go home."

TAKE REST!

It was time to practice. I stumbled to the top of my Yoga mat, came to attention, and thought, "Oh man, I do *not* want to do this." Lately I practice at 4 in the afternoon. I unroll my mat at the foot of our bed, on top of plywood sheets that I put down over the thick carpet. Yesterday, though, I was beat-tired. I had dragged around all afternoon, and even the thought of trying to fold forward was exhausting. Which leads me to wonder — When is it okay to *not* practice? When is it *advisable* to not practice?

In Ashtanga Vinyasa Yoga, we engage the physical, intellectual, and emotional levels simultaneously. Given the variables of those three branches, it's definitely possible to plateau, or even burn out. The Ashtanga Vinyasa practice in particular is physically vigorous enough that it's possible to experience many of the symptoms of overtraining, like fatigue, exhaustion, weakness, and depression.

I've never experienced true overtraining, though, because life, as is its wont, has hurled terrific curveballs at me, and I've invariably taken time off my mat, whether due to family obligations, work, travel, illness, or injury.

Let's say, though, that you've managed to avoid those influences that pull us from our mats, and also let's say that, for whatever reason, you've hit a place in your asana practice where you are stuck.

Maybe you can't perform equably the state of the asana, which most importantly in Ashtanga Vinyasa often includes the transition. Some of the more complicated asanas can take eight months to two years to perform as suggested.

My wife Tara took perhaps eight months to a year-and-a-half to comfortably address eka pada sirsasana. I started with Tim in 2001, and he adjusted me every single day in baddha konasana until I returned from India in mid-2004, at which point he said, "You no longer need my help."

Which meant I got The Squash five days a week for three years.

So what to do when you hit a pose at which you're stuck ... and a year slips past? And you're still on that pose, with no measurable progress?

First of all, allow me to repeat the old Yogic adage, "Practice non-attachment."

Man, that chestnut is bullshit.

"Practice non-attachment" has devolved into an empty cliché. It's turned into a yogic-New Age-Buddhist catchphrase. Usually it's uttered mantra-like as a result of pain that has arisen when a desire is not gratified or an expectation fulfilled.

You didn't get the raise you were expecting at work? "Practice non-attachment!" you tell yourself. The guy on the mat next watches you struggle to touch your toes in kapotasana and says, "Practice non-attachment!" This "mantra" helps you avoid looking at and experiencing disappointment, anger, sadness, and fear. It also creates a subtle sense of guilt and inadequacy, as though something were wrong with you for wanting to touch your toes in kapotasana.

And oh! If you only practice harder, more correctly, more fervently, then one day that glorious state of non-attachment will arrive. Then life will be one giant red-velvet cupcake with cream-cheese frosting.

Well, it's not going to happen.

Non-attachment is not a state or experience you can consume and enjoy. Attachment and non-attachment are two sides of the same coin. You cannot have one without the other. They are not separate. Attachment bounds, defines, and gives meaning to non-attachment. As soon as you try to "practice non-attachment" you are practicing attachment, because one can only ever exists directly opposite the other.

I don't want to utter a trite catchphrase as either deferment or deflection. Yoga doesn't teach me to defer my feelings and thoughts. It's not training me to detach or dissociate from them. It's teaching me to acknowledge them as they arise, see them for what they are, and then see that I am not those feelings and thoughts.

So, what to do? What to do when the plateau hits and frustration arises? Frustration is a normal part of a daily and intense practice. It sits side-by-side with intense effort. Intense effort is essential to getting up every day to get on the mat, after all. Like our friends "attachment" and "non-attachment," "effort" is not separate from "frustration."

It's helpful to me to know I'm not the first person to ever experience the plateau and its partner, frustration. Our friend Patanjali has some thoughts on the subject.

In book I, verse 30 of his Yoga Sutras, he addresses nine obstacles to practice. He calls them antarayah, or obstacles, and they function as citta-vikshepa. These obstacles scatter (vikshepa) the mind (citta).

The first antarayah he lists is vyadhi, which is illness or sickness. My practice of the Primary Series of Ashtanga Vinyasa strengthened my body and "purified" my mind and body of "toxins." I take purify in this sense to mean that my practice has made me more aware of my physical, social, dietary, and personal habits, and allowed me to tune, tweak or adjust all of them so I might be more effortless and more in tune with my life.

The second antarayah/obstacle that Patanjali lists is styana, or stuck-ness. Boom. Right away the second hurdle or distraction is stuck-ness. At a certain point, simply showing up daily and hurling myself at an asana didn't effect any further transformation on my nervous system.

Patanjali is helpful here, too, as he goes on to list in verse 31 some of the symptoms of the aforementioned obstacles. They should be familiar to anyone who's ever struggled with an asana: suffering or dis-ease (dukha), a sour or bitter outlook (daurmanasya)[13], anxiety (anga-mejayatva, anga meaning limb and mejayatva meaning trembling; this literally means shaking of the limbs), and an unsteady or arrhythmic in- and out-breath (shvasa-prashvasa).

Patanjali ends with the breath, thankfully, because while I can't practice non-attachment without practicing attachment, I can practice steadying and lengthening my breath (a technique Patanjali suggests in later Sutras), I can activate internal "locks," or bandhas, and I can then synch my movement to my breath.

If you've got a five- or six-day-a-week practice and you've hit a bumpy patch characterized by dis-ease, negativity, anxiety, and labored breathing, why not take time off? Stay home. Sleep in. Take a week or 10 days off.

I believe the longest I've been off the mat has been two weeks. This was while I recovered from knee surgery. Man, I really missed the practice. This experience led me to believe that if your practice is grounded and established, getting back on the mat will be the least of your worries.

Time off was also a very interesting exercise in observing the grasping or hoarding tendencies I had towards the practice. Thankfully, their scrabbling, clenching intensity diminished greatly after I noticed and named them. Sit and notice something and its power greatly diminishes.

Another approach I've enjoyed has been to practice as much or as little of the Ashtanga Vinyasa sequence as I could, which is often usually the standing sequence, and then sit. This required a ruthless appraisal of what I could and couldn't do, and has

---

[13] I like to think of the word "dour" or the phrase "crabby applesauce."

proved an excellent approach when I've been exhausted after travel, sleeplessness, or illness.

The overall idea here is not to abandon practice, but rather to reframe the idea of what an Ashtanga Vinyasa practice can be and should look like.

A constant practice-refreshing technique that Tara and I have tried to follow is to return every three or four months to see our teacher in Encinitas. So while frequent trips to a nearby teacher may not be possible, perhaps you might plan annual or semi-annual pilgrimages or odysseys to a retreat or intensive. You might even plan a trip to Mysore, India. Retreats or intensives are tricky, though, because they're easy to turn into ideals to be grasped and hoarded.

I don't want to just practice harder or more intensely. I want to practice smarter. To translate "practice smarter" to real-world, concrete principles is not easy, and it varies from person to person. For me, it's taken either the subtle artistry of a teacher, like Tim, or the commonsense perspective of a close friend, like my wife. Both give me a sense of perspective and scale. "Practice smarter" is more of an art than a science. This art is given shape and meaning by the boundaries of my own practice, my own reflections on yogic and other relevant texts, and my wife and my teacher's watchful eyes and helpful conversation.

So what did I do on that fateful afternoon, standing on my mat, facing our home altar, my first thought in relation to a Yoga asana practice the word "fuck?" Well, I honored that which I breathe, and that which breathes me, and then I served my body's immediate need for rest. I practiced one Surya Namaskar A, I sat down and breathed 25 ujjayi breaths, and when I lay down to take rest, I promptly fell asleep.

BLOG RESPONSE

I wrote the following in response to another person's blog post that questioned the methodology of a progressive, sequential sequence. I found that in writing it, I articulated and then revised many of my own thoughts regarding Ashtanga Vinyasa. I've once again revised it for inclusion here.

The first three series are progressive sequences. Over time, the later poses make the preceding ones easier, which might seem like good cause to skip ahead. It's very important to remember, though, that it is the initial poses make the later poses possible.

On a physical level (annamaya kosha), I've found Intermediate Series begins to seriously work with the plexus of nerves that runs through the sacrum. On a subtle level (pranamaya kosha), Nadi Shodhana begins to work on the kanda, the egg-shaped "knot" where the three main nadis, sushumna, ida and pingala, intersect; it also effects directly the sushumna nadi, which extends from the muladhara to the crown of the head. It goes to work on these areas with a series of progressively more intense backbends. After twists as counterposes and transitional resting postures, it then turns to the opposite direction with a series of intense forward bends. The Advanced

Series then flip-flop between more extreme directions with, shall we say, less compassionate transitions.

Pasasana begins preparation for backbending. Its twisting aspect continues the alleviation of forward bending that began with setu bandasana, and this pose begins to strengthen the back of the body as well as lengthen the calves. Subsequently, krouncasana continues to lengthen the top of the legs as well as the side of the extended leg. The following several poses all lengthen the connective tissue in the legs and, via backbends, the front core of the body. The peak is kapotasana, a very intense backbend.

After kapotasana, supta vajrasana helps reset the sacrum, and bakasana, which requires a rounded spine and sharply contracted abdominal muscles, continues the transition away from backbending. As a counterpose, bakasana strengthens the abdominal area, which when contracted will help support, lengthen and elongate the muscles of the back.

Bakasana is critical because this isometric support of the spine as well as the pelvis is essential once you've arrived at the first leg-behind-head pose. While it may be more challenging to do eka pada sirsasana than dwi pada sirsasana, the risk for injury in dwi pada is much, much greater, which is generally why it is given after some proficiency is demonstrated in eka pada sirsasana. Yogi nidrasana is aptly named, too. It's a relaxing, resting pose, and it begins the transition away from leg-behind-head, which carries through into tittibasana.

Tittibasana and karandavasana are counterposes to dwi pada sirsasana, as the spine is gradually brought out of the state of extreme flexion and the core is once again engaged to help return the spine and the muscles of the back to a sense of neutrality. Karandavasana also involves an intense rounding of the spine in order to fit the shins into the armpits, while the lift back up requires tremendous low-back strength.

The poses in Ashtanga Vinyasa and the arrangement of those poses can be more than just beads strung on the necklace of the breath, sequentially and linearly. The postures are at the same time recursive and nested within each other like matryoshka dolls, unique and individual yet at the same time containing the postures that both precede and follow them.

So rather than take the usual pose/counterpose dialectic, which is linear, chronological, and "arborescent," I find it helpful to use a triadic approach to asana sequencing. There's the attack, the ascension, the rising note, or the Brahma/creator aspect of the Trimurti. This aspect evolves into (and contains) the sustain, the plateau, or the Vishnu/preserver aspect. This is followed by the decay, the decline, dissolution of Shiva, the destroyer. Each is nothing but the other, and yet distinct and unique.

These sets or groupings create a third point between yourself and your object of regard, in this case between you and an asana, that creates perspective, scale, distance, depth, and therefore meaning and value.

For example, I could consider Baradvajasana the Brahma aspect of the leg-behind-head sequence, which culminates in dwi pada sirsasana, the Vishnu of the sequence. Yogi nidrasana begins the Shiva aspects of leg-behind-head. This perspective can create a sense of a wonderful liquidity as one asana flows into the next. It also creates different possibilities for relationships between and groupings of backbending, twisting, and strengthening.

It can be helpful to focus on the specific minutiae of the asanas, that hands must be bound, heels must be grabbed, et cetera, et cetera, although to borrow a phrase from Matthew Sweeney's *Ashtanga Yoga As It Is*, this is a phase through which one ought to move.

Concern with the rules, order and structure of the Ashtanga Vinyasa practice correlates to the Brahma or creator aspect, and over time must give way to the more mundane, workaday Vishnu aspect, and finally, into the whirling, artful Shiva-termite aspect, a practice that burrows into and devours its own borders as art and as an offering. As a long-time yogini once told me, "I used to be concerned about taking my heels. Now I just make the shapes." It's important to remember that, in order to move beyond a state of being concerned about taking her heels, she had to first experience that state.

The art of Nadi Shodhana, regardless of grabbing your heels or licking your coccyx, is to "make the shape," even if the shape is a fairly intense back- or forward-bend, while at the same time cultivating an ease-full, skilled state of observation and awareness. This state can be measured by a yogini's fluid entry and exit from the pose, her stability and calm (Patanjali's famous "sthira sukkham"), and of course, the quality of her breath, both the out *and* in-breath. This breath is ideally measured, even, and calm. Or, according to our friend Patanjali, dirgha and sukshma.

My pure speculation on part of the reasoning behind the way poses are given (or not) in Mysore is that Sharath can see a student's avoidance of a pose; for the most part, he's very practiced in reading a student's body and listening for the student's breath to determine their sthira and sukkham while they're in a pose.

This cultivation of calm, steady observation in a pose as stimulating as kapotasana both necessitates and is predicated on a retraining of the nervous system. The development of an unwavering internal candle flame is what I take Nadi Shodhana to mean.

It's not as important that, for example, one has to be lifted back up from karandavasana — though most everyone, given time and practice, can learn to place their feet in lotus and lower to their arms — it's the ease, fluidity, and most importantly, sense of non-separation from the process that's important. This is in itself a skill to be refined, learned and polished like a fine jewel.

There are many reasons why someone ought not to proceed through Primary without at least "making the shape," and chief among these reasons is injury. There is also a tendency to gloss over and ignore those poses we do not like or find difficult. Unfortunately, the sequences are progressive, though, so to skip something now is to pay for it later.

To use intermediate sequencing as an example, bhekasana is very important to kapotasana, as is laguvajrasana, among others. Until these two are not only comfortable but done correctly, kapotasana is very, very difficult. This is part of the reason why these backbends should generally not be given as a chunk or "sub-sequence." In fact, in my experience, kapotasana is incredibly difficult, indeed impossible, unless and until one can slowly and calmly lift and lower from standing into urdvha dhanurasana.

The desire to reach the next pose is a difficult aspect of this practice, but one that I believe many people, if not all, go through, and one that can be allayed through continuous, steady practice through all stages and phases of life — including injury, illness, and life-shifts.

I also find a triadic view of my practice and relationships in general as helpful. I have gone through Vishnu phases of practice, for example, when life demands meant I could practice an hour a day, 4 days a week. These were no less luminous than longer, more physically intense practices. The desire to feed my need for the next pose abated significantly in the face of life's ebb and flow. I was just happy to be on my mat.

Again, I thank you for your post. I hope my thoughts here help you reflect on your own practice, just as your post inspired me reflect on my own.

Best,
jason

BURN TO SHINE

Pattabhi Jois used to say, "Asana is correct, pain is going." Like Patanjali, Jois is nothing if not pithy. Notice that Jois does not say, "Asana is correct, pleasure is there." This is the same way the Advaita philosopher Shankara uses "neti, neti." In many respects, to use the affirmative to describe the state of an asana, as when trying to describe Brahman or the Absolute, is entirely inadequate.

Confusion arises when "feeling good" is conflated with the means and end of Yoga. "Feeling good" and Yoga often run parallel, but they are not the same pursuit. Quite frequently the practice of Yoga and the sensation of pleasure, not to mention comfort and ease, are entirely at odds.

The poet John Giorno wrote an autobiography called *You've Got to Burn to Shine*, and it's true. Sometimes, if you're lucky, your most deeply cherished beliefs get tossed on the fire, and the tapas of practice burns them up.

Sometimes that hurts.

THANK GOD FOR BOREDOM

The novelty will wear off. That is, the tyranny of the novelty of the Yoga asana will and should exhaust itself. Then the grim slog to the Yoga studio will become the most terrific aspect of the practice.

The days to treasure are the days of overwhelming inertia, the days when you have to manually lift one leg at a time in order to climb the stairs to the studio, only to unroll the same old mat in an empty, drafty room to practice the same sequence of poses you've done for years.

The inertia is a sign of something. Of what? Usually, when twitchy boredom arises, when my mind demands novelty and spectacle, inspiration and stimulation, the quietness that then arises during practice is deeper, richer, more resonant ... utterly boring and mundane and brilliant.

As Leonard Cohen said, when you give up the idea of creating your own masterpiece, the real masterpiece arises.

.

YOGA PHOTO DUKKHA

It wasn't until I saw photos of myself practicing Yoga asana that I became intimately familiar with the term "fruit basket." I'd purchased some tight blue Nike Yoga shorts (on sale) while in Tokyo. I wore them during practice, and then had my friend Kranti hoist me into kapotasana and shoot some photos. I'd always wanted to see what I looked like in the pose.

There it was: my bean-bag, shrink-wrapped in blue spandex, bulged prominently. This was the first time I'd ever had to consider my own fruit basket.

The revelation and obscuration of my coin purse was not a factor I had ever considered when I began to teach Ashtanga, which I came to through a gradual process of incremental nudges. Once the seed was planted that I might teach this style, it was watered a variety of ways, through conscious choice, the encouragement of my wife and friends, the support of previous teachers, and the occasional stroke of blind luck.

I feel very alive while "teaching" a Mysore class, that is, while sharing what was shared with me. When I began, though, I had no real idea of the full scope of what "teaching Yoga" meant in the Twenty-first Century. I'm talking about the fruit basket, but in a larger sense I'm talking about the Yoga Photo itself.

Through the practice of this Yoga, we "purify," collect, and direct our prana, both internal and external. I began generating small amounts of external prana by teaching at gyms, health clubs and Yoga studios, and these places began to ask for photos of me for Web sites or fliers.

These requests flushed to the surface my insecurity and fear about teaching. The decision to put myself out there in a picture was somehow significant. Was I worthy? Was I ready? Was I good enough? Did I have something to share? Did I understand this Yoga enough to pass along the technique? Ashtanga is a powerful and potent practice. I doubted my ability to awaken in every person the same feelings that it awoke in me.

Once I could articulate these doubts, though, they shrank as shadows in the noon sun. It's not the task of an Ashtanga Vinyasa teacher to deliver an experience. "Experiences" always and of necessity end. They're over as soon as class ends, at which time the Yoga is another experience consumed, categorized, and filed away.

I've noticed this tendency to consume Yoga writ large when it comes to traveling to practice in Mysore. I've had wonderful times in Mysore, filled with awakenings small and large, and of such intense sweetness that it aches to think of them.

I don't want to dutifully file away that time as "Awakening Experience," though. I could have chosen to return home to continually rehash that experience as my touchstone for the practice. I would then try to recreate that experience in myself, and worse, in the people who practice with me. Then I also pass along the idea that my experience from last year in Mysore is an experience to which everyone should aspire. All this while I anxiously await my *next* trip to Mysore to try to recreate this sweetness.

Not that I'm suggesting you shouldn't travel to Mysore! Or return there! I'm just suggesting to recognize the desire and tendency to turn an experience of connection, of Yoga, into an attainment, whether it's in a led class or a journey to Mysore. This is a disservice to my condition right now, whether I'm practicing on planks in my bedroom, in Encinitas, or in India.

Experiences come and go. A byproduct of the Ashtanga Vinyasa practice for me is that sometimes I clear up enough to stop identifying those conditions as myself. Sometimes I can even respond spontaneously, creatively, and intuitively to them.

I keep returning to a sentence from Tim's on-line biography, a line I have shamelessly plagiarized for more than 5 years: "My goal as a teacher is to inspire a passion for practice. The practice itself, done consistently and accurately, is the real teacher." From that perspective, teaching Ashtanga Yoga is simple: all I have to do is get out of its way.

Once my doubts about my validity as a teacher were addressed, or at least named and acknowledged, it became obvious to me that some sort of photo would be necessary. My practice of the Ashtanga Yoga system has led me to cultivate a deep appreciation for its maps of energy manipulation. I am serious about teaching this Yoga. Therefore I want to work with these energies in the most intelligent and skillful manner. If that meant taking photos, then so be it.

There are a host of issues that arise with Yoga photos. First, given the nature of digital media, photos are available at any time to anyone. Which means you have no say over the context or format in which people see them.

Second, the actual content of the photo is troublesome. Do you go for the 'craziest' asana you are capable of performing? Or something less threatening and more inviting? Do you try to look serious and profound, or lighthearted and personable? What if you can only hold the photo for the second it takes to snap the photo?

Then, of course, you must consider your wardrobe. Do you wear those skin-tight briefs you normally wear, or something more tasteful and concealing? And what about the setting? A Yoga studio? Indoors? Outdoors? Someplace exotic?

I imagine each teacher quickly arrives at the pranic budget they're willing to allot to thinking about this. There's a beautiful photo of Dena Kingsberg in kashyapasana, in which she's half-submerged in water, surrounded by forest. Or there are the photos of Eddie Stern, which don't seem to exist, actually, because Eddie clearly and consciously chose to not invest any energy in photos. For my part, I see no problem with wanting good, beautiful, and, one would hope, true photographs.

The most recent photos of me were taken by my friend Kelly Hubert. They work for me, and they're a conscious reflection of aspects of the practice that I value and therefore want to communicate. I like the colors, the asanas are nice and non-threatening, I'm wearing nondescript black clothing, and there's a shot of Guruji in the background. Done and done.

And this time, no fruit basket.

BOREDOM AGAIN

I get asked from time to time if I ever get bored doing the same asanas and the same sequences, over and over again.

I'm going to come clean about the Ashtanga Vinyasa sequences: for the most part, they are fucking difficult for me. Whichever sequence I'm practicing still demands the entirety of my concentration and breathing. Still, it's not that I don't occasionally juggle the sense of routine with the urge for novelty. Maybe I lack imagination or creativity.

Boredom is, though, in many ways a blessing, at least during the seated practices of pranayama and just sitting. For me, it signals that a certain part of my mind is rattling its cage for novelty and stimulation because it wants to avoid an impending quietude.

The question as to the boredom of a set sequence arises from people who have, I think, a fundamentally different conception as to the purpose of the asanas. Asanas can be therapeutic tools, they can make you fitter, stronger, more pliable, they can help you lose weight, and they can help you build muscle.

These two notions, that of asanas as fitness tools or therapy aids, are quite different from the sense of asanas as acts of devotional worship. If asana is the fourth limb of an eight-limbed plant, then asana is also yama, asana is also pranayama, asana is also samadhi. None of them are separate. However, as Pattabhi Jois has said about the eight limbs: "The first five can be taught. The last three can only be caught." I have taken that to mean that the first five are ones I can practice; the last three arise (or not!) as a result of the first four.

I'll give it another 10 years. Maybe at that point I'll have mastered the asanas, the transitions into and out of them, their sequencing, and the most skillful application of bandhas and drishti, in order to allow boredom to more fully arise.

MY LATEST PROJECTS

I'm writing treatments for several Yoga-related novels! They're gonna be squarely in the female romance-cum-memoir genre and they're aimed squarely at the beating heart lodged beneath the silicon-enhanced bosom of upper middle-class white women.

The Devil Wears Prana
A young Yoga teacher graduates from a Baron Baptiste Power Yoga Teacher Training and takes a job as an assistant to one of the world's premier power Yoga teachers. Shenanigans ensue as the young Yoga teacher struggles to cope with her boss' outrageous, bitchy personality and ridiculous requests. The Yoga world will be buzzing, I assure you, as it attempts to guess on whom the identity of the powerful Yoga teacher is based!

Yoga High School
After their guru takes mahasamadhi, a group of devoted teenage yogis and yoginis, with the help of Jai Uttal and the Pagan Love Orchestra, take over their ashram to combat its newly installed oppressive administration. Picture this closing scene: Yogis and yoginis twist and contort in various advanced asanas as the ashram burns to the ground behind them and Jai

and his merry bunch get all bhakti'd out on the front steps! I'll pitch this to the Weinsteins as *"Fame* meets *Rock 'n' Roll High School*— but with Yoga!"

Starve, Curse, Hate

The rebellion of no rebellion! The dropping out of dropping in! An upper middle-class white woman, tired of living a life of spontaneous, free-wheeling Yoga practice in a Yoga ashram in India, enrolls in college, obtains a law degree, and joins a law firm. At the same time, she falls in love, gets married, has children and helps maintain a family — all while engaging in a daily spiritual practice, as part of a living tradition and under the auspices of a teacher! This is pure escapist fantasy that's gonna hit every yurt-dwelling, granola-eating Burning Man yogini right in the chest-plate.

Ghee

This is the story of the yogini Martine, a young mother who arrives at a small, insular Yoga school in the Pacific Northwest with her 6-year-old daughter Penelope. Martine, a gifted cook, begins preparing and selling various dishes, all of which feature heroic amounts of the titular ghee. Her cooking siddhis begin to change the lives of the Yoga students through magic, which puts her in direct opposition to the school's guru, who sees Martine's use of siddhis as a distraction on the path to Self-realization. Salty tears will spatter your Lululemon top upon completion of this gem, I assure you! Though I trust that, if your top is Lululemon, it will wick away the moisture appropriately.

Sex and the Siddhi

This is gonna detail the intimate life of a sassy, raunchy New York City yogini who regularly meets her three yogini friends for lunch at various posh Hare Krishna temples in order to dish intimate details and eat veg samosas. Sample dialogue: "Then he manipulated my muladhara, I contracted my bandhas, and the kundalini rocketed right up my sushumna!" Titillation ensues. Each of the narrator's three friends is an extension of an aspect of her own personality, and together they function as her very own Trimurti!

SHANKARA VERSUS DOGEN

Shankara, as David Loy writes[14], had some very specific ideas regarding the usefulness of a Yoga practice: It is "for those of inferior intellect." Repetitive meditation techniques? They may be helpful because "people do not always understand the first time."

Shankara, or Adi Shankara, who perhaps lived some time around 800 CE, was the renowned scholar and consolidator of the strain of philosophy called Advaita Vedanta. In the world of Ashtanga Vinyasa, many who practice the Ashtanga Vinyasa pranayama sequence recite the first verse of the Advaita Guru Parampara to begin the four chants that close the practice. In so doing, they honor Shankara among the other prominent teachers of Advaita.

So it's a bit paradoxical to finish practice and then salute a preeminent teacher who didn't think much of "practice" at all. The *Brhadaranyaka Upanishad* (I.iv.7) suggests that "the Self alone

---

[14] "The Path of No-path: Shankara and Dogen on the Paradox of Practice," *Philosophy East and West*, Volume 38, Number 2 (April 1988), pages 127–146.

is to be meditated upon" — and Shankara does not agree. He comments on this line to say that "except the knowledge that arises from that statement ... there is nothing to be done, either mentally or outwardly."

Personally, I've found it useful to triangulate my relationship to a practice or belief-system with a third one, one that appeals to me and shares many similarities and yet also presents oppositions. It is this act of triangulation that helps me examine areas of overlap, areas of concordance, and areas of tension. I've heard Richard Freeman use the algebraic metaphor of the overlapping circles of a Venn diagram, in which one overlays different systems to see where they meet and, more importantly, where they don't. It is these areas where systems rub against each other that provide the richest, most useful insights.

In order to reconcile my practice of Ashtanga Vinyasa with its utter uselessness, at least according to a key philosophical figure in its tradition, it's useful to veer completely and totally in the opposite direction, and head towards Dogen, a key figure in the Zen tradition.

Unlike Shankara, according to Loy, "the heart of [Dogen's] teaching is this shusho itto (or ichinyo), 'the oneness of practice and enlightenment.'" More importantly, as Loy says, where "Shankara resolves the delusive dualism between means and ends by denying the need for any practice, Dogen resolves the same dualism by incorporating enlightenment into practice."

From this perspective, the limbs of Ashtanga Yoga are indivisible from each other. The practice of the yamas, the niyamas, the asanas, the pranayamas — the external limbs — are equivalent to the internal limbs — including, most importantly, samadhi. The practice of the yamas is samadhi; samadhi is the practice of pranayama. Samadhi is the practice of the asanas.

Loy's observations on the Zen practice of zazen echo Patanjali's famous "abhyasa vairagyam tan nirodha": "This does not deny the reality of enlightenment from the relative standpoint. Done in such a fashion — neither seeking nor anticipating any effects — zazen in itself gradually transforms my character, and eventually there is an experience in which I realize clearly that the true nature of my mind and the true nature of the universe are nondual. Zazen cannot be said to cause this experience; enlightenment is always an accident, as Chogyam Trungpa has said, but practice undeniably makes us more accident-prone."

ASHTANGA AND CROSSFIT

"Jason? Is that you?" Ben, an acquaintance from Near East Yoga, leaned his head into the gym door and squinted at me.

I was in the middle of a workout — to be precise, I was in the middle of a practice session — at Crossfit Portland. It's a typical Crossfit gym: there are pull-up bars along one wall, ropes and gymnastic rings hanging from the ceiling, and racks of barbells and bumper weight-plates.

A class was in the middle of a row/clean-and-jerk workout, so barbells were bouncing off the floor and people were heaving on the rowing machines.

Back in winter 2006, during Ashtanga Vinyasa Yoga practices, I tore the meniscus in first my right and then my left knee. So in spring 2007 I had both knees scoped, about a month apart. I had 25% of the meniscus scraped out of the right knee and 20% from the other. The surgery was ridiculously easy, as much as you can ever say that of surgery. I pretty much limped out of the operating theater within an hour of the 90-minute procedure, and two weeks later I walked down the aisle at my wedding.

The scarring, swelling, and stiffness lingered, though.

Meanwhile, for many years my close friend Nate had bugged me to try this thing called "Crossfit." Crossfit.com was a Web site that posted daily workouts, and Nate's older brother, a Navy

SEAL, had trained this way for years. They both swore by the system. People around the world would perform the workouts and then post their weights lifted and times recorded in the comments section of the site.

The workouts themselves were high-volume intervals that blended rudimentary gymnastics movements (push-up, pull-up, dip, muscle-up, air squat), the Olympic lifts, powerlifts, and anaerobic and aerobic work, such as running, rowing, or jumping rope.

Crossfit founder Greg Glassman had defined overall fitness as sustained power output, or "the ability to move large loads long distances over time," and the workouts were designed to increase this ability.

I wanted to do something to help heal and strengthen my knee, and I didn't know the first thing about working out on my own, so I took a group class at Crossfit Portland in fall 2007. At the time, the gym was just a small room in the corner of the Academy of Kung Fu in Southeast Portland.

I believe my first workout involved five sets of five deadlifts (5x5), followed by a workout called "Christine": a 500 meter row, followed by 12 bodyweight deadlifts, followed by 21 box-jumps, repeated three times as fast as possible.

I had done interval work and experience lung-death during hard chaingang road-bike rides before, so I was used to the lung-bursting aspect of the interval work.

However, I had never lifted a weight in my life, nor rowed, nor done pull-ups — any of it. I found that I liked it. More than that, I liked Scott, the owner of the place. Over time I've come to be great friends with him and the other owners, his wife Rochelle and Xi Xia.

They weren't jocks, they weren't aggro, they weren't meat-heads, and they weren't dicks — all associations I'd had since high school about sports, athletics, and athletes in general. If I hadn't loved riding a skateboard I would've been driven to it anyway, simply because I had poor experiences with high-school athletics, in that, at least at James Robinson High School in Fairfax, Virginia, the jocks were fucking douchebags.

I also greatly liked the community feel of the Crossfit classes. Everyone sweated, strove, suffered and triumphed together. There were no hamsters-on-treadmills-watching-TV as at the many gyms where I taught Yoga. It was a lot like a Mysore or led Yoga class: they touched the same desire for connection and conversation (or Yoga!) that we all have.

So, beginning in fall 2007 and until roughly winter 2009, I began practicing Crossfit two to three times a week.

An established and long-time Ashtanga Vinyasa Yoga practice really helped me in certain areas. I had an active, usable flexibility in many areas. It meant I spent less muscular energy on exercises like overhead squats, toes-to-bar, L-sits, or squats.

I had also always considered my shoulders and back "stiff," but practicing Crossfit in a group let me see just how much the concepts of "stiffness" and "flexibility" are absolutely and utterly context- and goal-based.

Basically, in Crossfit, flexibility was not a pursuit in and of itself. It was only a variable to be considered when practicing or performing a movement. This viewpoint coincides greatly with my appreciation for Ashtanga Vinyasa, in which flexibility is the means and not the end.

I also found I had a fair amount of proprioception, meaning I was able to pick up certain movements fairly quickly. As they say, "Flexibility breeds skill."

Unfortunately, as far as effort goes, greater flexibility and proprioception were irrelevant. To paraphrase three-time Tour de France winner Greg LeMond, "You don't suffer less — you just go faster." So although I was able to quickly figure out certain movements efficiently, and my flexibility meant I had much less muscle resistance, it just meant I could do more reps. I was still pushed to my limits.

When I say "more reps," don't mistake me. I was only ever a sub-par or mediocre (at best) Crossfitter. Towards the end of my Crossfit days, I was able to perform at least most of the bodyweight-only exercises with decent proficiency and mediocre times.

I finally worked up to several (but not all) workouts with the recommended barbell weights, such as "Diane," which is 21-15-9 reps of 225-pound deadlift and handstand push-ups, though I want to say my best time for that was 10 minutes. Many guys typically do it in 3 or less.

I feel like I had a good sense of how to regulate, lengthen, and employ the breath for whatever effort was required, whether it was a short, sharp explosive exhale in a max-effort lift, a rhythmic in-out during lots of push-ups, or a deep belly breathing between rounds to help bring down my heart-rate in order to recover. These techniques didn't always work or work well — part of the point of Crossfit is to push you to the point where your systems break down to expose weakness. So don't misunderstand me: the workouts could be hard and grueling.

Years of smooth and steady breath-movement vinyasa had also utterly detrained my fast-twitch muscle fibers. I had to relearn and practice any explosiveness or speed. Both my wife and I did these ridiculous slow-motion burpees, absolutely at odds with the purpose of the exercise.

Finally and quite obviously, the most glaring lack of carryover from a Yoga practice was an utter lack of strength. I could handle most of the bodyweight exercises okay, as when I started, I weighed in at a near-starved 140ish pounds. However, when it was time to move a fixed weight, I was a total novice. I was weak.

The press, the back squat, the deadlift, the snatch, the clean and jerk: I began all of these as a pure beginner, with entry-level weights. This was humbling because, as most of us know, Ashtanga can be hard, tiring, and sweaty. I often left the Yoga studio and felt I had just worked hard.

Unfortunately, there was no carryover.

Ashtanga did nothing for muscular endurance, either. All these years of chaturanga dandasanas did not carry over in any way toward performing 20 push-ups, for example.

Also, years of daily pranayama might've expanded my lung capacity, but it had done nothing for my use of that lung capacity. Meaning, I still struggled during intense bursts of strength and after 500-meter rows or 400-meter sprints. I speculate that a seasoned Ashtanga Vinyasa practitioner can perform several of the Ashtanga series with their heart rate at between 100 and 120 beats-per-minute. So it was absolutely revelatory for me to back-squat a heavy weight 10 times, drop the barbell, then sprint for 400 meters, my heart-rate pinned at 180. To use a subtle energy-body map with workouts like that, they opened and used radically different nadis than I had been accustomed to.

Crossfit provided some great benefits, too. It greatly aided in rehabbing my knee. I strengthened and supported all the muscles, ligaments, and tendons around, above, and below the joint. I felt that Bulgarian split squats, back and front squats, single-leg deadlifts, and standard deadlifts really helped.

The Crossfit system tends to pair exercises that work complementary muscle groups. The workouts are generally arranged to work different energy systems as well, which let you work harder and longer than if it had been related muscle groups. For example, a pull exercise is paired with a push, and then followed by a low-body heart-stopper such as box-jumps or sprints.

The system also favors exercises that strengthen the posterior chain, as in back, glutes, and hamstrings. I believe exercises built around both of these principles cleaned up a couple small but persistent injuries. Specifically, kettlebell swings and glute-ham raises (GHRs) really sorted my low back.

In a much larger sense, Crossfit helped me realize the true importance that strength plays in health, longevity and performance. I got a bit stronger and I felt better, both during Yoga practice and just walking around. Of course, I've also gained 15 pounds.

Crossfit really made me appreciate the various active flexibility components built into the Primary Series. For adults, merely increasing your passive flexibility is not the smartest, safest, or even efficient way to become more "flexible." The key, which is a by-product in the intelligent application of the Primary Series, is to get stronger and more flexible at the same.

The practice of Crossfit also led me to greatly appreciate my own unique cycles of effort-adapt-recovery. I began to notice this cycle in my own asana and even pranayama practice. Crossfit training worked best when it followed the following classic formula: build a foundation or base, follow it with hard efforts, then reduce or back off. This always resulted in super-compensation or break-through.

That formula as transposed to traditional Ashtanga would be: accumulation, or to work "pose by pose" or "one by one"; intensification, or the addition of a new pose; and finally, reduction, or Moon Day, weekend, or holiday.

This explained why I frequently felt stronger after a few days off.

I don't have a perfect application of these principles to the Ashtanga practice, but understanding them has led me to better understand and work with my energy levels and experiences on the mat.

Still, Crossfit didn't help the Ashtanga practice in all ways.

I would feel immediate loss of range-of-motion (flexibility) during and after some of their notorious high-rep or high-rep and loaded movements. For example, after "Angie," which is 100 pull-ups, push-ups, sit-ups and squats for time, my pec minor and pecs in general really shortened to the new range of movement. After any workout with thrusters (a barbell front-squat push-press) my hip flexors would noticeably shorten and my Hanumanasana depth decreased. I personally have never been an immediate and gifted back-bender, so I had to be diligent about maintaining that area of flexibility. Often I would intend to practice backbends after a Crossfit workout, but this didn't always happen, often because I was so smashed.

The fatigue from three or four Crossfit workouts a week often added a richness and depth to my practice. This fatigue, delayed onset muscle soreness (DOMS), and neural drain forced me to reframe why I practiced Ashtanga as well as how I could practice it when I couldn't lift my arms over my head or walk up a flight of stairs, let alone practice an entire sequence.

The relationship between Ashtanga Vinyasa and Crossfit was reciprocal. The practice of samyama, or dharana, dhayana, and samadhi was possible during the short and intense workouts, though not as much during 20-minute or longer workouts.

Certain Crossfit skills, once learned, were simple enough that I was in no danger of muscular or aerobic failure, and the workouts were short enough and timed, which meant I couldn't dissociate from my body, as I've experienced on long bike rides or runs. Attention was immediate and total. Concentration would subside into contemplation, and absorption would arise. During some workouts and then immediately after there would be the experience of a luminous clarity.

My good friend David Kennedy laughed when I told him that I really liked the flush of health and vitality that accompanied back-squatting. "You think the only way to wake up kundalini is to wear a turban and do funny breathing?" he asked.

It's like, duh. If God is *in* all things *as* all things, then of course a universal and pervasive energy isn't tied to a specific cultural or physical techniques.

Don't tell the Kundalini Yoga people, but that energy arises under a barbell as well as it does performing ustrasana or bhastrika breathing.

Another huge revelation I had during hard efforts was the immediate and somatic confrontation of fear, of failure, and of the unknown. Personally, it was revelatory to gaze over the edge of absolute muscular and aerobic shut-down.

This to me is similar to a Yoga practice. Not that in Yoga we barf on our mats from the effort! At least, I don't. No, it's more living with an emotion or thought long enough for it to wear thin and be exposed for what it really is: an emotion or thought.

Some of the workouts also dramatically expanded my horizon as to what I consider difficult, even what I consider possible. I used to consider the limits of physicality the Sunday led Intermediate series class in Mysore and at Tim's Encinitas studio.

Spending time under a barbell, though, or doing a "Full Mission Profile," or any of these other "mental toughness" workouts really expanded my sense of what was really "difficult."

They drove home one of Pattabhi Jois' constant points: "Body not stiff. Mind stiff!" A lot of my perceptions of my abilities turned out to be just that — perceptions.

These workouts and this training really made me okay with doing what I could do. During a 100-percent effort or a max-effort attempt on a barbell lift, often there was literally nothing else physically I was able to do. That was absolutely okay. I put forth honest, sincere effort, and then let go. I simply tried to never quit. To paraphrase Krishnamacharya, "Do the Yoga that can be done!"

Eventually, though, by winter 2009, I began to lean into my passions and interests and away from Crossfit.

Once I learned the movements and the novelty wore off, I realized there was also a routine to it. I didn't have an event or activity to train for, and without that, Crossfit was just a numbers-collecting game: add one more pull-up to my max, 10 more pounds to my press, 10 more pounds to my deadlift, ad infinitum.

On the day Ben poked his head into Crossfit Portland, I wasn't actually doing Crossfit. I was doing my recent physical practice, of which I'll write more later.

I wrote this for two reasons. The first was because, some days after Ben saw me, his girlfriend asked my wife Tara, "Does Jason ... *work out?*"

The novelty, minutiae, and exhilaration of the Ashtanga Vinyasa sequences can be profound, stirring and all-consuming.

It's important to remember, though, that the asana sequences are not the be-all, end-all of physical expression and/or personal devotion.

I also found Crossfit to address fundamental physical, emotional, and psycho-spiritual needs that the Ashtanga Vinyasa practice and culture either ignored or disdained.

The first of these needs was pure physical exertion. Ashtanga Vinyasa is derived from Smarta Brahmin culture, and so there is a veneer, however thin, that physical exertion is lower caste and class. Group physical exertion also opens the door to competitiveness, aggression, and anger — but also absorption, ecstasy, compassion, and empathy.

In Ashtanga Vinyasa Yoga culture, and in Yoga culture in general, we seem intent to play up those latter qualities while ignoring the former, even though they are a fundamental part of human experience.

My understanding is that one of the many questions that Ashtanga Vinyasa Yoga asks is not "How can I get rid of aggression, anger and competitiveness?" but rather, "How can I savor, use skillfully, and work with those qualities, as they are not me?"

So I'm thankful I was exposed to Crossfit. I'm tremendously grateful for the friend's I've made through it.

It has also really made me appreciate the beauty, subtlety and simplicity of the breath-movement that is Ashtanga Vinyasa Yoga. It's fun to leap around like a spastic monkey, but the breath-work and the internal focal points, as well as the connection to people of the same interest, are what draw me back to my yoga mat.

YOUR UNIVERSE

I saw the following on John Gruber's Daring Fireball blog this morning:

> "Stanley Kubrick in his 1968 interview with *Playboy*:
> 'The most terrifying fact of the universe is not that it is hostile but that it is indifferent; but if we can come to terms with this indifference and accept the challenges of life within the boundaries of death — however mutable man may be able to make them — our existence as a species can have genuine meaning and fulfillment. However vast the darkness, we must supply our own light.'"

I submit that what Kubrick refers to here as a "fact" — that the universe is inherently "indifferent" — is nothing more than the meaning he himself has ascribed. I also suggest that we can expand out Kubrick's perspective to view three possible perspectives, postures or "seats" (asanas) one can take on the universe:

1. The universe is against us.
This is the belief that the forces of the universe are deeply inimical, antithetical, or opposed to our desires, dreams, and very

being. I have known people like this in my life (for example, my own brother) and have, at times embodied this view myself. Ah, the teenage years, when I thought (in alphabetical order) that Bierce, Bukowski, Camus, Celine and Sartre, among others, had figured it all out, and were offering the best way of thinking about my life. There is a victim mentality that seems to accompany this posture. This asana reminds me of Abel, of Cain and Abel fame, a story that, among other things, tells us that there are predators and there are victims. One of life's questions then becomes, which one are you?

2. The universe is indifferent to us.

Kubrick's quote above is typical of this view, though it seems to me there's underlying this asana is the idea that the universe is in fact a "vast darkness." It also seems this view is typical of what's considered the modern Western materialist view — that the universe is reducible to tiny components that inhabit a separate space through which we move. This theme also seems to thread its way through much of the Vedas — that the universe is comprised of eating, and eaters, and we're all just a link on a food chain. On a mythic level, I think of Sisyphus: we are here to roll the rock up the hill again and again, an inherently futile effort, yet one in which we must find beauty and meaning.

3. The universe supports us.

As emanations of the universe, the "one turning," we are in fact not and never separate from everything else. From the perspective of this asana, we are here to move in synchrony with and to participate in it. In this way a Yoga practice becomes the practice of not freeing ourselves from life or overcoming it. Ram, Sita and Hanuman embody this: conditional love, unconditional love, and the agent that re-unifies them, each moving according to their capacities, desires and duties.

I think it's important to know how your system of Yoga addresses these postures, as each one does so differently. To look at these three views as asanas is helpful, as the image of a consciously chosen seat implies personal choice and the power of our intention and attention. Which of the three views do you choose to invest in, knowing that in turn, this view will inform and infuse your life?

I think it's also possible to hold opposing seats at different times, too. What situations cause fluctuations in your asana? Family, work, relationships? For example, how does spending an afternoon at the DMV (to choose one of my favorite examples) affect your asana?

To return to Stanley Kubrick: his perspective, that of the vast indifference of the universe, infused his films, from *Dr. Strangelove* and *Barry Lyndon* to *The Shining* and *Full Metal Jacket*. So while his films are among those I respect, admire and am moved by, I find I can't love them like I love Truffaut (and not Godard), Renoir, Pasolini, and Anderson (Wes and Paul).

MY LEAST FAVORITE POSE

Everyone has one posture that they absolutely dread. For me, it was baddha konasana. That pose hurt. A lot. I couldn't put my knees down. I couldn't really sit up, but then I also couldn't move forward. It was this painful limbo. And I was confronted with it, every single day.

I went to Home Depot, bought two empty sandbags, and filled them with sand from Moonlight Beach. I would get up every morning, put a sandbag on each leg, and watch CNN while drinking my morning espresso.

Now, years (and years) later, I quite enjoy the posture. What happened?

There was a gap, a blind spot, between where I wanted to be, where I thought I *should* be, and where I was. The dread came out of that gap, a gap that was a disconnection or disunion.

The pose was painful, difficult, and frustrating. I craved the dramatic fireworks of release. I hoped one day that an emotional and physical elation would overtake me when my knees and chest finally hit the floor together.

It never came, of course.

Baddha konasana was for me a slow, steady polishing of perhaps three years. One day I could breathe, go forward, and become absorbed in the breath, the spine, the hips, the belly and navel, the tongue against the top teeth. The sound of my breath swelled and receded in my chest, I was flat on the floor and goddammit, it was no big deal.

The beautiful limitations of practicing an imperfect sequence of postures, as they all are, as in Ashtanga Vinyasa, is that there will always be another posture to spark friction between the calcification of what ought to be and the fluidity of what is.

Dread or fear is one of the residues of lingering in calcification, one I'm pleased to say is avoidable. The simple, practical physical technique that facilitates a return to what is, to *this*, to *this*, to *this*, is quite simple: inhale, exhale.

To strive to perform an asana to the exacting and impossible standards of a fixed, graven image in my head only threatened to break me. Perhaps the shards would have been beautiful, but the pulling, straining or spraining of muscles, ligaments, and tendons, is not what I consider Yoga.

Mind you, I think it's important to work hard. It's important to have standards to give shape and direction to my efforts. It's important to show up and give my best each day. It's equally as important to be pushed as restrained.

But it is impossible and disingenuous for me to force my personal Sunday second series practice to replicate the led second series class in Mysore, and I know this because I have tried. To try to do this is to ignore the given conditions of reality as it is at that moment.

So while I light candles every single morning to both Pattabhi Jois and Tim Miller, and they are both responsible in part for every inhale and exhale I take, I have worked hard to get Guruji, the icon of the man, off my mat.

Yes, he was stern, he was demanding, and he wanted us to work hard, but my interpretation of his teaching is that, when we left Mysore, we were to take a living practice with us. We were not to reduce this Yoga to the worship of a memory of a man in Mysore. "Everywhere looking, God," he would say, and that means looking now, and not backwards at some experience in the shala from 10 years ago.

As I continue with this practice, I've noticed that my self-illusions and tendencies don't go away. I'm not sure I'd want them to, either, though I can recognize them now for what they are: illusions, preferences, and tendencies. Like Rumpelstiltsken, once named, they don't seem to have such power. The skill of the yogi is the skillful manipulation and enjoyment of those tendencies, and perhaps even the realization that those illusions are gifts to be skillfully shared.

When I returned to the Encinitas studio from my first trip to India, Tim padded over to me as I prepared to take baddha konasana. He glanced down and shrugged.

"Well," he said, "I guess you don't need me anymore," and walked off.

Of course, my revelatory postures continued predictably from baddha konasana to backbends, to standing from backbends, to kapotasana (Oh, kapotasana …). Over time my appreciation has grown for these opportunities to experience friction. It is still a very real practice to stay with my breath and my bandhas.

My god, kapotasana put me through the wringer, and still does, and there are so many more to come … Hanumanasana, supta trvrkrmasana, trvrkrmasana. It never ends.

I hope it never does.

HOW TO GET SIX-PACK ABS WITH ASHTANGA

There's a scene in the documentary *Ashtanga NYC* in which a woman smiles, a cat with the canary in its mouth, and says, "Well, we all know Ashtanga can give you a great body!" This said as if the particular brilliance of Ashtanga Vinyasa is that we can be spiritual *and* have washboard abs.

I certainly experience the desire to look good naked. Enmeshed within this desire, too, is the idea that the harder I work or exert myself, often physically, the greater the sense of spirituality or connection that will arise. In other words, in order to reap the greatest benefits from Ashtanga, I really need to feel the burn.

I still experience the occasional relapse into that mode of thinking when I confuse causation with correlation. Often, after I've undertaken an intense Yoga asana and pranayama practice, I leave the studio suffused with a grounded yet buoyant clarity, as well as a sense of at-home-ness in my own body that seems to emanate from the very DNA in my cells. I often mistakenly think this sense of well-being is *caused by* the amount of effort I put out. It's then an easy leap to think that if I put forth *more* effort, I'll get even *more* in return.

It took a couple years to realize that this "equipoise" was the residue of practice itself, and would either arise, or not, regardless of the amount of sweat I left on my mat. This realization only occurred as a result of life's inevitable vagaries. There've been instances due to relationships, work, illness, or injury that I could only practice partial sections of the series, for example standing and finishing, and it was mind-blowing to realize this "equipoise" would arise after a only short 20-minute practice, a sequence that entailed linking the ujjayi breathing to simple compound movements, taking a seated posture, and then taking rest.

Still, I wouldn't trade in the "work harder" mentality. It's fertile soil from which deeper relationships can develop. This "work harder" mentality is what drew me to the mat and helped me nurture a consistent Yoga practice, and it dovetails with the rules-oriented stage of learning the Ashtanga system, which is when the specific minutiae of the vinyasa and the general philosophy behind it become of vital interest.

There is an occasional, aw-shucks acknowledgment of the physical transformation this practice, coupled with dietary changes, can create. It has a difficult Primary Series that we are initially expected to practice 6 days a week, and this can and will transform one's body in many ways, just as it transformed and continues to transform mine.

When in my early 20s I undertook a committed Yoga practice and began to pay attention to what I ate as well as how to embody my own body, the Ashtanga Vinyasa practice wrought changes large and small. I believe it's important to not only acknowledge but honor the desire to look good naked, the desire to feel beautiful, and the desire to feel at ease in one's own skin.

The shadow aspect of this and any hatha Yoga practice or physical discipline: narcissism. Thankfully we are not the first to confront these issues. Far from it. In the *Yoga Sutras*, Patanjali is very clear to balance disciplined practice with self-study and devotion.

I don't practice Yoga to eliminate or extinguish desire, or as a means transcending my own life. I've also never met anyone free from desire, and I've never met a saint. Desire makes life possible, after all, and there's a great argument for the idea that life is desire.

I find the practice of Yoga helps me clear the confusion of my desires and preferences with my essential nature. It doesn't mean I don't have desires and preferences. It's just that practicing samadhi means my desires and preferences don't lead me around.

To layer on guilt for having the desire to look good naked, or for having any thought or desire, really, turns this or any practice into an insidious means of self-torture.

Desires arise. Thankfully we have simple tools, like the tristana that allow us to watch them, and by watching them, disempower their frenetic immediacy — perhaps even employ those desires skillfully.

YOGA TEACHER CONTRACT RIDER

As those who read my weekly column "Yoga Hustla" know, I have my left hand grasped firmly around the throat of the Yoga world. There is not the slightest tremor on Indra's many-jeweled net that is not picked up and published by yours truly. Even as you read this, I'm working my other arm around the head of the Yoga world in order to put it in a crushing sleeper hold.

So doubtless all will be as excited as I am with this week's veritable treasure find — the contract rider of one of the world's biggest celebrity Yoga teachers! A contract rider accompanies a performing artist's or celebrity's contract to appear in public, and includes specifications on stage design, sound systems, lighting rigs, as well as the artist's wish list, from transportation and billing to dressing room accommodations and meals.

What does this big-time Yoga celebrity, whom I shall call "YOGA TEACHER" for fear of both legal and physical retribution, require to show up at your shala to teach the kids downward dog? And who could it possibly be? I'll never tell, so read on, o yogi …

YOGA TEACHER RIDER AGREEMENT

This rider to the contract date _____ by and between YOGA TEACHER (hereinafter referred to as "THE ARTIST") and _____ (hereinafter referred to as "THE YOGA SHALA") for the engagement is made part of the setting-forth of additional terms and conditions to attached contract.

A. One LARGE BASKET of WHITE FLOWER PETALS (any genus) to be strewn at ARTIST'S feet during the "Grand Entrance." (Shala owners responsible for clean up.)

B. One NEW LARGE MANDUKA BLACK MAT, to be laid at front of Yoga class, to be surrounded by AMBER-SCENTED CANDLES and wiped down with scented SANDALWOOD OIL.

C. Photographs and videos will be allowed in special "MEDIA AREA" to be set up facing ARTIST'S LEFT SIDE. Also, all photos or video must be approved by ARTIST'S PUBLICITY AGENT.

D. Pyrotechnic requirements during ARTIST'S bandha demonstration to be paid for by shala owners and to include:
  1. One smudge pot
  2. Three M-80 firecrackers
  3. Smoke machine with dry ice

E. Workshop accommodation requirements include a dressing room separated from main Yoga shala by a door with lock (henceforth to be referred to as "VIP ROOM.")

F. TOUR MANAGER to be supplied with five "VIP PASSES" to permit entry to "VIP ROOM."

G. At ARTIST'S discretion, select workshop attendees may be invited to "VIP ROOM" for specific and individual manual bandha adjustments.

H. VIP ROOM craft services table to include:
1. One bowl of M&Ms. All red M&Ms to be removed!!! [Sic]
2. One vat Tiger Balm, large
3. 12 bottles de-ionized, charcoal-filtered, glacier-drip water served at room temperature
4. 6 unbleached organic hypo-allergenic cotton towels with thread count of 500 or greater
5. One large bowl (two cups) brown rice
6. One bowl steamed veggies, to include broccoli, chard, burdock root, carrots, beets, kale
7. One extra-large bag of chocolate-chocolate chip cookies
8. One extra-thick bar of Toblerone dark chocolate

I. Workshop organizers will arrange an autograph signing to take place immediately after workshop and not to exceed 15 minutes.

J. Questions NOT TO BE ASKED of ARTIST at any time during workshop:
1. "Are you Certified?"
2. "Are you still teaching Madonna?"
3. "Can you do kapotasana?

PAIN, SUFFERING, ET AL

I'm sorry to report from the front lines of a Yoga practice that Ashtanga hasn't created for me a pain-free or even a suffering-free life. Thus far there's no sitting in lotus and floating blissfully above the tidal pull of life's glorious little catastrophes.

I make an important distinction between "pain" and "suffering." Pain is a reflex reaction, a signal to withdraw from pain-causing stimulus. Suffering tends to be thoughts and thought-patterns associated with that pain-causing stimulus.

Ashtanga gives us the tools to help clearly perceive this aspect of suffering. This practice is not designed to relieve us of pain, however — though it's not designed to cause us pain, either, despite what other Yoga teachers say. (So quit wrenching your leg into lotus!) The effect of physical pain relief through injury rehabilitation is but a secondary effect of the Yoga. The practice of Ashtanga provides several tools to cultivate the practice of clear perception: the union of a breathing technique to movement, several internal focal points, and the cultivation of the discipline of a daily practice.

All of which are designed to create a specific understanding on a somatic level: My suffering is caused not by specific sensations, but by my thoughts associated with those sensations.

This realization is the tip of a deeper understanding that I am not, in fact, the sum total of these or any thoughts.

I've found that Ashtanga has given me the tools to see with great precision and clarity exactly when my thinking is causing me suffering. Often this suffering arises during the states of the asanas themselves, or transitioning between them. For example, some days, a posture will feel much, much harder than it did the previous day, or when I was younger, or when I was uninjured.

My thoughts usually go like this: The physical stimulus is registered, whether it be stiffness, discomfort, or perhaps pain. Next, it is cataloged in comparison with a previous experience. Finally, I link a judgment to that comparison: "This sucks," or "This should be easier," or "This was easier last night," or "Why doesn't this feel like Friday night's class?"

Kaboom! Instant suffering. Reality and my expectations of reality have inevitably failed to match up.

The trickier aspect of suffering comes when the asanas are enjoyable or pleasurable. As they say, it's easier to root out the thorn than spit out the honey. It's easy for me to bask in the sensory pleasure of the endorphin rush of a full series. But even this is merely setting the stage for future suffering, because my next practice, and the next one, and the one after that, will now invariably fall short of this internal mental benchmark.

So what to do? The human mind has evolved to organize and catalog, weigh and measure. The Indian goddess of worldly illusion is named Maya, which is derived from a root meaning "to measure, demarcate." I don't feel that this measuring, this Maya, is something or someone to suppress, overcome, silence or eradicate. Attempting to do so only gives the mind more to weigh, measure and catalog.

This is where the return to the fundamentals is critical: vinyasa, bandha, drishti. Practiced correctly and consistently, these techniques are simple and powerful enough to allow to arise observation of the maelstrom of the internal dialogue. I find that when I observe something, I don't participate in it, which somehow robs the experience of its power.

It's not that thoughts won't arise, nor that I'll stop experiencing emotions — the Yoga is not a narcotic, after all — but their immediacy, their seriousness, gradually loosens its iron-clad grip.

HOW TO DO ASHTANGA AND CROSSFIT

This is written from the perspective of someone practicing a full sequence (and change) five to six days a week.

1. Eat More
Food and nutrition are highly personal and emotionally charged practices and beliefs.

This suggestion isn't about the content of your food, however, whether it's vegetarian, vegan, omni, or what-have-you. It's about quantity.

I've had conversations with lots of people who practice Ashtanga Vinyasa and, y'know, I've been around for a couple years, so I've seen how some Ashtanga Vinyasa yogis and yoginis eat.

If you commit to Crossfit a couple times a week, you are going to need to ratchet up your food intake. This is usually not a problem because you will be ridiculously hungry after doing both.

I only have one suggestion as to what you should eat if you do Ashtanga Vinyasa Yoga plus Crossfit, though it's more a suggestion of what *not* to eat — processed foods.

2. No Really — Eat More

By "eat more," I don't mean an extra bowl of popcorn, an extra spoonful of cottage cheese, more yogurt, or an extra banana.

You're going to need to put away some protein, fat and carbohydrate in order to recover from your efforts *and* support your future practices.

3. Sleep More

At least nine hours a night. Seriously.

This is usually not an issue because you will be tired. You will need the sleep.

However, you will dig yourself into a hole if you try to slide by doing both Ashtanga Vinyasa and Crossfit (plus work, family, happy hour, pranayama, meditation, puja) on six hours a night

4. Off Days Are Off

Saturdays and moon days are opportunities for reflection and relaxation. Do nothing.

5. Less Flexible

I'm not going to sugar-coat it for you: high reps plus reduced range of motion (ROM) means your nervous system will shorten muscles accordingly.

You will get less flexible by doing hundreds (*Hundreds?* Yes, hundreds.) of pull-ups, push-ups, squats, thrusters, dips, muscle-ups, et cetera, et cetera.

Good thing we are not practicing Yoga to get more flexible, right?

…

Right?

… anybody?

6. More Strength

Maybe you trade off a bit of flexibility — for a period of time. You will, however, get stronger.

If you've never done resistance training, like I hadn't, you will get a shit-ton stronger.

Your maximal strength, strength-endurance, and endurance will increase (though these last two will diminish when you stop practicing Crossfit).

7. Enjoy Yourself

Ashtanga Yoga's not so hard. Neither is Crossfit.

I mean, they're both challenging, and some days are like a warm, effortless shower and some are like a root canal, but that's not unique to either discipline.

A serious-as-death attitude doesn't help, either on the mat or in the gym. Plus those people aren't that much fun to be around.

So go ahead and enjoy yourself, both on the mat and in Crossfit.

WHITE ELEPHANT VERSUS TERMITE PRACTICE

Manny Farber was one of the most important critics in movie history, a legend who penned classic pieces for *The New Republic*, *The Nation*, *Art Forum*, and *Film Comment*. He was an early champion of the American action film, as well as of Hollywood stylists like Howard Hawks, Don Siegel, Sam Fuller, Preston Sturges, and even Chuck Jones. He's most famous for the essays "Underground Films" and "White Elephant Art Vs. Termite Art."

In the latter piece, Farber introduced and championed what he called "termite art," a phrase he coined to describe any unpretentious movie that "goes always forward eating its own boundaries, and, like as not, leaves nothing in its path other than the signs of eager, industrious, unkempt activity."

He contrasts this termite or tapeworm film to what he termed "white elephant art," or "masterpiece art." This was art that was "artificially laden with symbolism and significance." The white elephant films of Michelangelo Antonioni, for example, "pin viewers to the wall and slug them with wet towels of artiness and significance."

What might characterize a white elephant Ashtanga Vinyasa Yoga practice? Perhaps we could say that dramatic, histrionic flourishes coupled with a promiscuous ujjayi breath might characterize a white elephant Yoga practice, as each vinyasa and each asana flashes with seriousness and "significance." A key characteristic of white elephant art, according to Farber, is that it's filled with "overripe technique."

In contrast, the termite practice is laconic, workmanlike, efficient; a termite practice, as Farber defines termite art, "nails down one moment without glamorizing it, but forgets this accomplishment as soon as it has passed." The termite practice is epitomized by an economy of expression.

To engage in a termite (or, as Farber elaborates, a "tapeworm-moss-fungus") practice, as the very name suggests, is to concern oneself with a burrowing into the many layers of the self, each layer as fine as onion skin, and not peeled so much as enveloped, chewed, swallowed, and digested, until one is left to confront the paradox of the self-devouring uroboros, the ancient Greek depiction of the snake or dragon eating its own tail.

You will not notice those termites at your studio as their economy renders them invisible. They will arrive, practice, and depart without drawing your attention. A termite's practice is entirely separate from physical ideas of flexibility and strength; it is compact and internal.

Among the ways to cultivate the termite aspect of one's practice, as Matthew Sweeney suggests in *Ashtanga Yoga: As It Is*, is to practice alone for an extended stretch of time. An unintended benefit of the solitary termite practice, as those around the world who practice alone know, is the deep and overwhelming sense of gratitude that arises from deep in the core of the body.

On a mundane level, a termite practice favors the rooting and grounding of the out-breath, while the white elephant practice favors an upward and expansive in-breath. The key difference is that both sides of the termite's breath are directed internally, while the white elephant's prana is drawn upward and outward and dissipates externally. In this regards, Yoga studios with mirrors run the risk of developing white elephant practices as the mirrors pull the prana to the surface.

The stereotypical white elephant inhales and exhales with thunderous momentousness, and each movement up and down, forwards and backwards, is rigid with overwrought concern for perfection. It is a practice over-burdened with floating fireworks and a concern for rubbery circus flexibility. The white elephant is entirely dependent upon the strict division between the practitioner, the practice and, most critically, the sense of spectators who view the practice.

Fortunately, it is this sense of performance that transmutes the white elephant. While "on stage" and acutely aware of the gaze of others, the white elephant activates and engages each and every body part in a steady diffusion of consciousness.

So there is value in the white elephant practice as, true to its name, it inevitably lumbers inward: the relentless focus on the performance and perfection of each asana, and the interlocking vinyasa between, can only lead the white elephant to dissolve in the performance. Any sense of separation between performer, performance, and audience dissolves entirely. One thinks of Shiva's aspect as Nataraj, whirling through his never-ending dance of destruction and creation. The dancer, the dance, the audience: all are one.

Who does not begin practice as a white elephant? Who does not enter a new studio or workshop as a white elephant? A key characteristic of the white elephant is its own self-consciousness, and who has never felt self-conscious? Whose practice does not flip-flop between white elephant and termite stages, sometimes even in that infinitesimal gap between the inhale and the exhale? The transition from white elephant to termite comes as one continues to practice: thoughts arise, one observes them, and one returns to the breath. One must "over-ripen" and become rotten with technique before sinking, diffuse, back into the mud and loam of a dance offered for its own sake.

MYSORE FLASHBACKS

My alarm is set for 4:03 AM, but I always wake minutes before it goes off. Somehow my body anticipates it. Often I drift back to sleep.

Sometimes, though, I lie awake and smell the crisp pre-dawn air and listen to the early hour's utter stillness, a stillness that reaches from my flat to the universe beyond.

In that hazy early hour, as sleep is slow to recede, Mysore comes back to me, charged with oneiric energy, my memories stronger and starker than possible during waking hours. I often just get image splashes:

A pre-dawn scooter ride to the shala, cotton-swab clouds soaking up spilled-paint oranges, purples, and pinks. The chill cuts through my sweatshirt, and my hands are cold on the plastic handlebars. The streets, normally full of people, animals, cars, motorcycles and rickshaws, are wide and deserted.

There was a tiny puppy up the block from our house on a 6-inch leash. The leash-end is weighted to a pile of gravel by a single cinderblock.

Another puppy lived around the corner from the house. She would follow me for three blocks as I walked to the shala, then three blocks as I walked home. The puppy grew to a dog right before my eyes. One day she doesn't follow me the three blocks home because she's stiffened in the ditch by the road, dark bloated body sharp against grass so green it hurt the eye.

The trip to the river, when we swam out to the rock crusted with dried bird shit. Everyone so careful not to put their heads under the water! We sunned and laughed and talked, there in the middle of the river. Everything clear and perfect. I could tell these strangers anything, only there was nothing to tell because it was all in front of us. Everything was right and true, and this was as perfect as life could be. For the lift back to shore we hopped into a passing coracle, an inverted hat woven from thick bamboo.

I piss on roadside rubble during an emergency bathroom break. I am not as hidden as I thought and a passing truckful of workers cheers. I wave one-handed and decide against embarrassment.

The spongy, manicured grass at Lalith Majal, decadent on the bottom of my feet.

A small sign stuck in the ground at the Southern Star hotel reads "Every seed a longing."

There are more visitations and hauntings from this time, too, some so beautiful and pure they're painful to reflect on during the day. I often think, "Was that me? Did I live that life? Was I that person?" Sometimes Mysore seems so very far away.

Something happened there, something more than consumption or vacation, something more than even the practice of Yoga asana. A way to be with none of the accumulated trappings of the "me" that have built up over the years. A sloughing off of the habits, routines, and expectations that had fixed in amber the ideas of "I" and self.

My alarm fires at its appointed time and flushes away the last of these visitations. I know when I go back to Mysore it won't be the same. I never visited this Mysore, because this Mysore never existed.

The love remains, though. I chisel and polish, heat and cool my heart to keep it open.

LIVING TRADITION

This was written before Pattabhi Jois passed away.

Ashtanga Vinyasa is a living tradition. Both parts of that phrase "living" and "tradition" are important considerations.

It's "living" in that we're fortunate enough to have Pattabhi Jois still living and (mostly) teaching in Mysore. The system grows, changes and evolves as he sees fit, one hopes based on his years of experience practicing, teaching, and observing.

In this regard, I consider his book *Yoga Mala* a manual, one to which serious practitioners should give serious consideration. However, I also try to bear in mind that that *Yoga Mala* was first published in 1957. I personally would not want to be treated by a doctor whose most recent medical texts and techniques came from 1957.

Many fundamental techniques and concepts about medicine and anatomy, as well as vinyasa, bandha, and drishti, have not changed since 1957. They have, however, evolved.

Ashtanga means "eight limbs," after all, and not "eight stairs," "eight steps," or "eight rungs," and implicit in the word "anga" is the conception of a system that is organic and interrelated.

As a tradition, Ashtanga Vinyasa is comprised of established techniques and sequences, and is best transmitted by a teacher and then practiced in a prescribed manner. There are many benefits to practicing within a tradition. It's vital to me to have other people, a teacher or otherwise, tell me, in effect, "Hey! You're not the first to experience this. I've been there, I've felt that, too. Now get back to your breathing, bandhas, drishti."

This is helpful beyond advice on how to press your lotus into handstand or grab your thighs in a backbend. A friend of mine has been teaching Mysore-style Ashtanga for many years, and he maintains that charisma is the first siddhi to appear from a sustained Yoga practice. When the siddhis manifest, a teacher and tradition will ground you. It means having a community to remind you not to nail your students. In my case, when Hanuman spoke to me during breathing practices, it meant I had someone tell me to focus on my bandhas, and when I walked out of the shala, suffused with Oneness, it meant someone reminded me to take my shoes.

So if you abandon the confines of a tradition — and they are confines, make no mistake — and follow your inner guru, you hold up the mirror to yourself. What tends to happen? At least in a Mysore room, I've noticed that practices begin to play up the practitioner's strengths and avoid their weaknesses. It only serves to sharpen one's sense of a separate self.

When you hold your own mirror, you open yourself to various blind-spots, pitfalls, and subtle but pervasive and very powerful tendencies. In a similar way, Narcissus held up his own mirror. In the Hellenic version, he leaned forward over a river to admire his own reflection and then fell in and drowned. In the whirlpool of conditioned existence, one would imagine.

Do you "need" a hands-on teacher, as opposed to, say, practicing from *Yoga Mala* or *As It Is*? Or Richard Freeman's or Sharath's DVD? Of course not. You don't need to live in Spain to learn to speak Spanish — though it sure can accelerate the process.

Then there are the questions as to the legitimacy of the manual you're using, and which texts you choose to pay attention to. Many of us who practice Ashtanga Yoga in the West aren't deeply embedded in a specific culture and faith, and so don't have texts we consider scripture. This has freed us to practice Yoga, though the shadow aspect is that, as we're ultimately free to choose our own scripture, we're able to cherry-pick texts that support our tendencies, desires, aversions, what we want to believe, and what makes us feel good.

For me, *Yoga Mala* is a practice manual, and supports my practice. It creates a perspective for context. It and other texts remain incidental and secondary to the practice, though.

More important than texts, a good teacher also holds up the mirror. I'm grateful for my teachers, who prod me when I'm lazy and cuff me about the head when I take pride in my practice. The different Ashtanga series can serve as teachers of their own. They are (relatively) unchanging and ever-present, and it takes discipline to get up every morning to perform the sequences. But then, it takes even greater discipline, one might say heroic discipline, to surrender to them.

It is so very difficult to abandon the notion that I always know what's best for myself. Often, perhaps usually, what's "best" for me tends to be what's pleasurable or self-satisfying. It can become fantastically difficult to discern when I'm operating from self-interest when aspects of the practice begin gratifying subtler, deeper psychological notions of self.

The key seems to have been surrender, though this surrender is also a practice for me, too, one enriched by love and faith in both a teacher and the teachings.

HOW TO START A MYSORE PROGRAM

My experience practicing and transmitting this style of Yoga has been a continual reaffirmation that to learn the Ashtanga Vinyasa sequence, one posture at a time, the postures and pace suited and scaled to each person's physical and mental conditions *at that very moment*, is the best way to teach a Yoga asana practice.

Look, we can get into the issue of whether the Primary Series is the most ideal sequence for that person, and we can also get into the shadow aspects of the Primary Series, as well as the implicit assumptions and belief structure woven throughout ... but *this shit really works*.

Here are some tips and suggestions for anyone interested in starting a Mysore program in their neck of the woods.

1. Get A Space

To find a satisfactory space is very tricky. This might be the *second* most difficult part of hosting, holding, facilitating or, god help me, *teaching* Ashtanga Vinyasa in the Mysore style.

A lot of people just rent a storefront or warehouse space. This means signing a lease as well as a series of other issues with which I have no experience, such as parking, insurance, renovation, maintenance, front desk and employee management, retail, etc., etc.

A lot of the older Mysore studios in the States were in shadier or run-down neighborhoods, simply because floor space was cheap. The Ashtanga Yoga Center in downtown Encinitas, It's Yoga in SOMA in San Francisco, Yoga Works on Third Street in Santa Monica, Ashtanga Yoga Los Angeles in Los Feliz and then Silverlake, Ashtanga Yoga New York, as well as tons of others. Some of those places stuck around long enough to watch their neighborhoods gentrify.

I practiced with Noah and Kimberley at their first space, on Sunset in LA. It had cement floors onto which I poured heroic quantities of sweat. I believe the place had been a hair salon or barber shop, because when I left I had 8 pounds of hair trimmings glued to my mat.

The actual physical requirements for a Mysore space are small, though, so you could conceivably rent anything because all you need is a room. Thank god we practice a style of Yoga that doesn't require elaborate props like these wall-and-belt contraptions I've seen, as well as elaborate blocks, bolsters and blankets. Sure, the props are helpful, just not a necessity.

The best yoga prop I use is an old fold-up massage mat donated by a long-time practitioner. The only prop I would ever install is a Swedish ladder or Stal bars. We have at Yoga Pearl, where Portland Ashtanga Yoga is hosted, stacks of various blocks. I'm not averse to using them as the situation arises, though I don't see them as essential.

So if you want to rent your own space, you can sign the lease. You might want or need to put down a wood floor, which would then be the main expense.

There are other ways to find studio space, though, some of which might more organically serve the current needs of your community, which, let's face it, might be five people. I've practiced at many different places during my global vagabondage. Maybe some of these locations might ring a bell with you.

Yoga studios are the obvious go-to. Once, when I traveled to Michigan, I rang the local studio and paid a drop-in to use their space during an open slot. It's not a far cry to then offer to rent or sublet the space each morning to hold Mysore class. You could arrange to pay a monthly fee for Monday-Fridays, 6 to 8 or 7 to 9 a.m.

My only suggestion is pick whole numbers for your class times, and then be as consistent as possible. Time slots like 6:15 to 8:45 on Monday, Wednesday, and Friday, then 7 to 9:05 on Tuesday and Thursdays, are confusing as hell. Personally, I strive to be as inclusive as possible, but within the boundaries I've established. People agree to take me on as an asana and pranayama technique teacher, but it's a two-way relationship in that I choose to assist them, too.

There are quite a few other places I've practiced that would work as a Mysore space: Pilates studios (we moved the "reformer" machines out of the way each morning), climbing gyms, boxing gyms, martial arts studios, dance studios (the mirrors are always a bummer), the Sandcastle Room and the buffet room at the Encinitas Best Western (cigarette smoke in the carpet in the former, breakfast crumbs in my mat in the latter), living rooms and bedrooms from Encinitas and Portland to Tokyo and Mysore, of course, as well as on the enclosed rooftop on Monica's house in Auroville.

Regardless of dirt, mosquitoes, carpet, mirrors, or croissant crumbs, hopefully the space is warm, safe, and available daily.

2. Let 'Em Know

I have the firm conviction that everyone can practice Ashtanga, though not everyone will *want* to practice Ashtanga in the Mysore style. People come to this practice as though coming home to a long-lost friend. Those people need to know about it.

The obvious outlet is the Internet. Do not waste your time or money with print ads. Register a web-site for $10 on Google Sites or get a free blog site, and put up the particulars: time, location, cost, maybe a brief description of what you offer and of Ashtanga Vinyasa and the Mysore-style.

Get a Facebook group going. You could also try Craig's List. It's free, so why not? (I've never done this, so let me know how it goes.) For meatspace promotion, you could always flier New Age bookstores (if you've got one) as well as coffee shops.

Finally, maybe the most important detail of all: if you've attended teacher trainings or workshops, tell everyone with whom you attended that you're hosting a space.

In fact, tell everyone you know, period. Word of mouth is huge.

3. Show Up Daily

This may be the most difficult part of hosting a Mysore space. Constancy is the queen of kings. Constancy is also gnarly. But to grow your community, you've got to show up every day, or as you've scheduled. Be present with the people in the room. Be active. Be engaged, whether there're two people or 50.

As a teacher, a Mysore class hums and crackles with more people than fewer. However, I always feel that regardless of how many turn up to practice — and I've taught Mysore class with 2 people and with 65 — these people woke up early, established their intention and their commitment, turned up at the studio, and unrolled their mat(s). I try to meet that intention and commitment with my own. Just something to be prepared for.

4. Seriously — Show Up Every Day

This is not a workshop, a retreat, or a hobby. A Mysore class is every day. Be ready for that! It's also an additional physical demand. In my case, I move around constantly for three hours a pop. So physical burnout is a real issue. I watch out for a key symptom of physical over-reaching, which is mental and emotional fatigue. I can tell when I'm frying out because my desire to get on the mat evaporates.

I define "over-reaching" as when my physical output outstrips my recovery. The one-on-one exchange of energy in a Mysore setting can be intense and, if you're not careful, enervating instead of innervating.

I also have my own Ashtanga Vinyasa practice that I tend, as well as other physical pursuits and interests. I try to be careful when I dial up the intensity of each, and I try to get enough sleep and eat enough food. My personal strategy thus far has been to plan or program chunks of time away from the studio once every month or six weeks. This is a process, though, and not a fixed schedule. The moon days really help, and I try to plan a trip if the moon days fall on several Saturdays.

I also think there's a lot of value if you can offer a Mysore class Monday thru Friday, or even Sunday through Friday, although I know conditions vary.

5. Stick To Your Guns

The longer I've done this, the more I've come to appreciate that it's the rules, boundaries and limitations that we agree on that add depth, value, and ultimately meaning to our practices.

I teach Ashtanga pose-by-pose because I've seen again and again that it's the best, safest, most approachable way to learn it.

If someone is interested in exploring their own sequence or another style of yoga, there are other studios in Portland that are better suited to their needs. I believe this system works best for almost everyone, so I try to explain it to them in this way. If they're interested in practicing, great. If not, then, as I said, there are other studios that can help them.

6. Remember Why You Practice

It's been helpful to me to articulate and then re-articulate why I practice Ashtanga Vinyasa Yoga in the Mysore style. This "why" is not inorganic and inert, and has grown, evolved, expanded and deepened over the years. I have the sense this depth and breadth as a result of the practice is an infinite process that will never finish, complete, or close itself off.

This process of examination and re-examination is what keeps me energized and interested, so I recommend finding ways to lean into your own interests, Yoga and otherwise, so that you can bring them back to the Mysore room with vigor and vitality.

Some people lean so hard into other pursuits they end up leaning away from Ashtanga Vinyasa, which is okay. Just be clear when that happens.

Personally, I practice Yoga for connection and intimacy, with myself and my own breath, and with other people who want the same.

I find most other systems of Asana-related Yoga to be overly pedagogical: a teacher stands up front and inspires while the class makes different shapes; often there's music playing. This setting can be fun and can spark us to practice, but ultimately our experience is only transmuted and reframed by our own deep practice. This deep practice has to be one's own practice, and one's own practice thrives when aided and abetted, not by an inspirational figurehead delivering sermons from the mount, but from someone who nudges, pokes, and grunts at us in various ways and on a daily basis.

In this regard, the Mysore-style setting is among the most profound because we do our own deep practice with a teacher and with each other.

7. Discover Why You Teach

I can often see in others flickers of what I consider samadhi, or delighted absorption. Sometimes a detail I provide helps someone reframe their experience of self, perhaps providing greater depth. Often this is the result of ridiculously mundane verbal cues, physical taps, or even base grunting. These experiences are infinitely rewarding for me.

I also love talking about this shit, so it's nice to have a community of people with whom to discuss the nuances of the philosophy.

8. Do Your Own Practice

This is the trickiest aspect to hosting a daily morning Mysore practice. I do 6-9 a.m. at Portland Ashtanga Yoga; I have spent time in Japan hosting a program that ran 7-10 a.m. In Encinitas, Tim has opted for 7-9 a.m.

In other words, if you start a morning program, you will most likely give up your morning practice.

I have friends who practice at 4 a.m. before their Mysore classes, and I have acquaintances who used to rise at 2 to begin practice at 3. So it is possible to commit to a daily morning practice and teach Mysore-style.

Personally, I found it thrilling to practice at 4:30 or 5, though the resultant asceticism became a merit badge, and turned early practice away from upasana or devotion and more towards self-gratification. My hermetic tendencies ran rampant. To wake retarded-early to practice meant I could say no to a social life. The sense of not needing anyone or anything is intoxicating, and I thrived on this sense of power and control over my life, and in fact over life itself.

Still, that period ended, and in fact was only possible during a period away from Tara and Rowan. I enjoy hanging out with my family and participating in — and thereby supporting — my culture (in other words, fulfilling my dharma), and so while I've explored early-morning practice, I'm not currently served by it. I want to put my kid to bed at 8, and not the other way around.

This was just my experience at that time. I suspect now an early morning practice would be different, simply because I would only practice that early if was that or no practice.

Without the energizing presence of a Mysore community around it, my physical practice has changed quite a bit, too. It's softer, slower and often bears a different flavor of intensity.

This is a detail to be prepared for, and will be a shock if you still live for those come-to-Jesus asana practices.

9. You Must Hate Money

Perhaps your financial issues are sorted (employed spouse, inheritance, investments), but starting a Mysore program can be lean times in the beginning. Mysore programs are like gardens and require daily, consistent, patient effort. Even then, you might perhaps end up serving four or five people.

I've heard it said to expect roughly 10 people per year, and that's if you aren't a total mouth-breather, have a good location, show up consistently, and tell people about it. So 4 years, 40 people.

The picture gets grim when you start your studio or program and realize it's very difficult to balance banker's hours with a daily Mysore program and your own practice. This means a traditional "career" can be a challenge to maintain. How are you going to maintain your marketing, P.R., banking, or programmer job if you can't network at conventions or happy hour, stay late at the office, or hit it early to make the phone meeting with Europe?

It is the 21st century, though, and there are tons of off-site, reduced hours and telecommuting jobs that pay well and require less than the traditional 8 hours per day. Plus there are many smart yoga teachers who seem to handle their finances in a smart way; Pattabhi Jois himself definitely enjoyed the prosperous aspect of his studio.

ABOUT THE AUTHOR

Jason Stein has practiced Ashtanga since 1998. He lives with his wife Tara and daughter Rowan in Oregon, where he currently owns and directs Portland Ashtanga Yoga. He conducts Mysore and led classes as well as workshops and retreats in the U.S. and internationally. To set up an event, contact him at leapinglanka@gmail.com.

This is his first book of personal work.

For more information, please visit leapinglanka.blogspot.com or portlandashtangayoga.com. Twitter feed @leapinglanka.

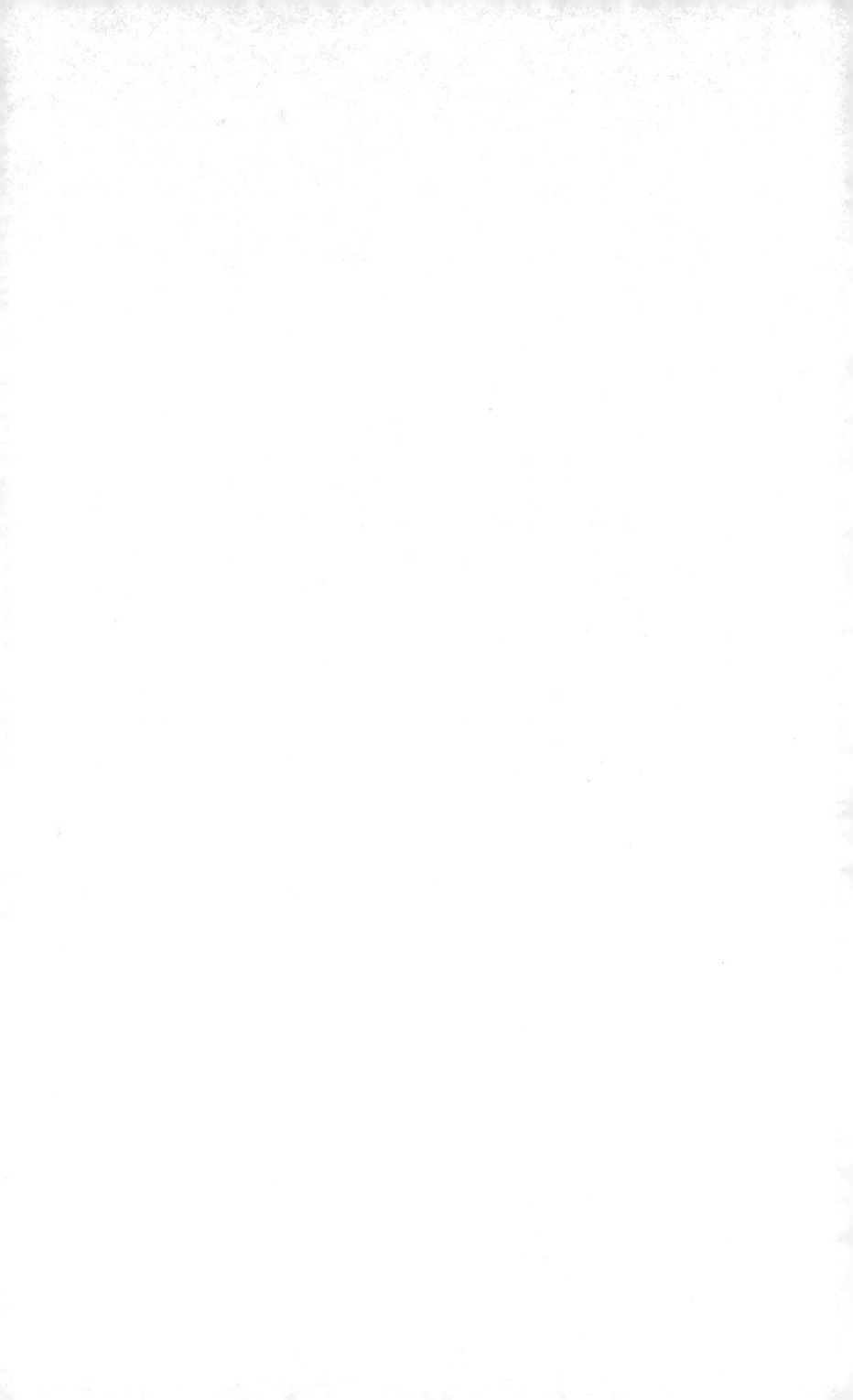

Made in the USA
San Bernardino, CA
18 November 2015